YOGA FOR
MIND, BODY & SPIRIT

Yoga for Mind, Body & Spirit

13-Digit ISBN: 978-1-64643-092-5
10-Digit ISBN: 1-64643-092-1

This book may be ordered by mail from the publisher. Please include $5.99 for postage and handling. Please support your local bookseller first!

Books published by Cider Mill Press Book Publishers are available at special discounts for bulk purchases in the United States by corporations, institutions, and other organizations. For more information, please contact the publisher.

Cider Mill Press Book Publishers
"Where good books are ready for press"
PO Box 454
12 Spring Street
Kennebunkport, Maine 04046
Visit us online!
cidermillpress.com

Typography: Agenda and Amatic SC
Image Credits: All photographs used under official license from Shutterstock.com.

Printed in China
1 2 3 4 5 6 7 8 9 0
First Edition

YOGA FOR
MIND, BODY & SPIRIT

*Poses, Meditations &
Wisdom for Leading a
Balanced Life*

CIDER MILL
PRESS

BOOK
PUBLISHERS
KENNEBUNKPORT, MAINE

Contents

Introduction

Yoga nourishes more than your body. The teachings that inform yoga have ancient roots in building a strong sense of self, creating contentment in the present moment, and providing a space and method for us to connect with our bodies. This is why yoga is the most effective when it is approached holistically; it was never meant to be reduced to a workout. Moving meditation engages our physical, emotional, and spiritual selves, providing us with a way to integrate the many versions of ourselves that we are forced to separate to keep up with the often hectic energy of our world today.

The ultimate form of self-care is not what looks glamorous or simply what feels good. Instead, it is a commitment to growing and nurturing all levels of your being, even when that requires difficult work. This book will provide you with a framework for multiple forms of self-exploration. Taking time to move through these mental and physical exercises will push you to engage with yourself in new ways, creating new connections between your internal self, your body, and the life you lead.

The first section of this book delves into the history of yoga. Before you head to your mat, explore the traditions behind this sacred practice. Understanding what influences our modern perception of yoga will give you a perspective into how this practice can ground the body while elevating the mind.

The second section is organized into 52 contemplations; you may wish to read one contemplation per week and use the week to explore how these ideas and concepts resonate in your daily life. Alternatively, you may want to flip through and find a contemplation that interests you. If you're feeling called to it, then chances are that is an area where you may be drawn to explore your thoughts and feelings. You can always return to this rotation of contemplations and challenge yourself to continually expand your awareness and thoughts, drawing on the lessons you've already learned to deepen your spiritual connections.

Following these contemplations is a series of step-by-step instructions to help guide you through a wide range of poses. All of them are accompanied by a helpful illustration to help you envision the motions and form of each stretch. You can work through these poses based on the order in which they appear, poses that help you access similar emotions, or poses that stretch and strengthen specific areas of your body. You can try a new pose every day or get a refresher on your favorites whenever you need it. This comprehensive guide is made to provide you with all of the tools you need to move into these poses with confidence. Mixed throughout these poses are several series of pages with inspiring imagery and encouraging quotations. Allow these to serve as a spiritual connection as you work through the poses.

The last section of the book, Practices, contains a series of yoga flows that you can try out. These allow you to stretch multiple muscles and work through emotional blocks by combining specific poses that "flow" into each other. You can select a specific practice that suits your situation and energy, or open to a random page for an impromptu experience. These practices are usually 5 to 15 minutes long, but feel free to shorten them by taking fewer breaths or skipping poses, or lengthen them by putting a couple of these short practices together. This is all about what works for your body and spirit. You never have to overexert yourself. When you're ready, you can always challenge yourself to do more. You can also use this book as a reference for individual poses, or to create your own flow with targeted stretches for your body. Through practice, you will learn what feels right for your body and what areas you may need to work on.

You will be able to return to the exercises in this book, both physical and spiritual, throughout your life. Whenever you need to release tension, open your heart, or connect with your highest self, yoga and its teachings will be there for you. You can go through this book in order or choose a pose or contemplation that calls to you. Whatever you do, know that there is no wrong way to use this book.

A (VERY) BRIEF HISTORY OF YOGA

FOR THOUSANDS OF YEARS, yogis have been asking, "Who am I?" and "How can I be happier?" For most of its history, yoga has not been an exploration of physical practice, but rather a deep and devotional inquiry into the depths of human consciousness.

Yogis have wrestled with such questions as:

▶ Who am I?

▶ What is my purpose?

▶ What is my mind?

▶ What is my soul?

▶ Is God separate from this world?

▶ What is suffering?

▶ How can I experience a life of liberation and freedom?

Yoga philosophy is part of one of the oldest continuous cultures on the planet: Hinduism. Hinduism is an umbrella for the wide array of schools and philosophical ideologies that evolved in India over the last several thousand years. Like a great tree, Hinduism has many branches. However, although many of the philosophical schools of thought have different practices or ideologies, they are all oriented to two central questions:

"Who am I?"

"How can I be liberated from suffering?"

Yoga is one of the branches on this tree.

Throughout its history, Indian culture has tended toward inclusion rather than suppression. Competing philosophical schools were more prone to debate than domination. This attitude allowed divergent schools of thought to flourish and evolve over time. The different philosophical schools of Hinduism called *darshanas*, or "viewpoints," and their variety demonstrate how each philosophy can provide a different way of looking at the same thing.

"The Blind Men and Elephant" story is a metaphor for this outlook. According to the tale, village inhabitants had never seen an elephant before. When an elephant arrived in their village, they ran to their local wise men, all of whom were blind.

Each blind man felt a different part of the elephant.

One felt a tusk and said, "Ah, it's like a rhino!"

One felt the tail and said, "It's like a horse!"

One felt its sides and said, "It's a great wall!"

One felt its trunk and said, "It's a snake!"

"There are hundreds of ways to kneel and kiss the ground."
—Rumi

The wise men were in complete disagreement about what the elephant really was because they each only had one part of the story. From a different perspective, however, each wise man was sharing the truth. Although their perceptions were different, they each were expressing an aspect of the truth.

Applying this story to the philosophical schools of Hinduism, we can see that no point of view would discredit another; each simply has a different access point to the truth.

There are six "orthodox" schools of Hinduism that trace their origins back to the Vedas (the oldest Hindu texts):

▶ Samkhya

▶ Yoga

▶ Nyaya (logic)

▶ Vaisheshika (atomism)

▶ Mimamsa (interpretation of the Vedas)

▶ Vedanta ("end" of the Vedas)

There are also three philosophical schools that do not cite the Vedas as their scriptural authority and are categorized as "unorthodox":

▶ Buddhism

▶ Jainism

▶ Carvaka

Like siblings, these different philosophical schools have grown up and played with one another, exchanging ideas like sisters might trade clothing. However, unlike the other schools, Yoga tends to focus on practice—rather than theoretical understanding—as a means to liberation and insight.

The umbrella of Yoga covers a wide array of different philosophies and practices. If the Yoga tradition is one branch on the tree of Hinduism, it is a branch with many offshoots and variations.

The origins of Hinduism are shrouded in mystery, but many scholars trace its roots back more than 4,000 years to the Indus Valley Civilization. The Indus Valley Civilization emerged in northwest India and Pakistan, where several ancient cities sprung up along the Indus and Sarasvati Rivers.

The earliest texts of Hinduism were composed during this time. The Vedas, from the root word *vid*, which means, "to know," are the first sacred Sanskrit texts. The Vedas are considered *shruti*, or "revealed wisdom," which means that they were created by humans, but were channeled from a higher source through divine insight. The Vedas include a variety of texts, including ritualistic chants delivered by priests. These early rituals were likely shamanic in tone, and used sacrificial fires and precise recitations to appease the gods and ensure that the natural and social order ran smoothly.

One of the last additions to the Vedas was a group of texts called the Upanishads. The Upanishads are also considered shruti, and are revelatory stories and contemplations emerging from the ecstatic (and perhaps intoxicated) state of its practitioners. These contemplations are metaphysical in nature and look deeply into the nature of self and identity. The Upanishads emerged from the meditations of groups of ascetics who fled society to retreat into the forest and focus on their personal liberation. You can almost envision these practitioners as ancient hippies who left society in order to pursue countercultural spiritual practices.

Upanishad means "sit down near," likely reflecting the close relationship between the guru (teacher) and student. Interestingly, although the earlier chants of the Vedic priests were used to uphold natural law and order, the writings of the Upanishads are intimate in nature. These meditating ascetics were far more interested in personal spiritual liberation than in upholding social norms. although the Upanishads are in one sense an extension of the philosophical insights of the Vedas, they also mark a radical departure in thought. The external rituals that characterized the Vedas became internal rituals of self-mastery. Rather than offering fire sacrifices to the gods, the ascetics instead sacrificed their attachments to ego, society, and worldly pleasures to experience divine insight.

The Upanishads gave birth to many of the core concepts that formed the foundation of Yoga philosophy, including the *prana* (energy), *karma* (the residue of cause and effect), the role of the guru, and the practice of meditation as the path to enlightenment.

The wisdom of meditative insight became crystallized in *The Yoga Sutras of Patanjali*, composed around 200 CE. This text is a series of short aphorisms that details the workings of the mind and outline practical tools that support the pathway to yoga, or liberation. This text illuminates the complexity of the mind's workings and provides practical tools to support practitioners on their spiritual journeys. As in the Upanishads, practitioners were advised to leave the distractions of society and avoid all sensual pleasures (including relationships, meat, and alcohol) in order to achieve liberation. Living a spiritual life required fasting, abstinence, and worldly renunciation.

Fortunately, for those of us who aren't interested in living in remote caves, Yoga philosophy evolved to include "householders" (people with family, living in society). The Bhagavad Gita, composed more than 2,000 years ago, made yoga accessible to everyone by offering new paths for practice that did not require worldly renunciation. A thousand years later, tantric philosophy revolutionized the practice, declaring that the world (and therefore the human body) was the expression of divine consciousness. With this new perspective, the material world was no longer an obstacle to spiritual liberation, but a living expression of divine consciousness. This world-positive viewpoint opened the door to a range of new tools that leveraged the sensory world as a pathway to spiritual liberation, including subtle body practices, sound, and mantra.

From the bosom of tantra, hatha yoga emerged as a philosophy that expanded the use of body-centered practices (including breath practices, cleansing techniques, and *asana*) as tools for practice and liberation. Several hundred years and a trip across the ocean later, and we now find ourselves practicing yoga postures and breath control as a means to control the mind, reduce stress, and increase our general well-being.

TEXTUAL REFERENCES

For our philosophical concepts, we will primarily refer to two different texts from the Yoga tradition: *The Yoga Sutras of Patanjali* and the Bhagavad Gita.

Composed around two thousand years ago, these texts contain many of the essential ideas that inform the Yoga tradition and our practice today.

The Yoga Sutra was compiled around 200 CE. Although authorship is attributed to a sage named Patanjali, this may be a *nom de plume* for different contributors. The name Patanjali literally means, "fallen offering," suggesting that this text was received from heaven as a gift. Sutra means, "thread." The book is a series of short, concise "threads" that could be memorized by students. Each thread encapsulates ideas and wisdom that could be the further subject of discussion and interpretation. *The Yoga Sutra* summarizes the key insights of the *jnana* (wisdom) Yoga tradition, which used meditation as its primary tool for spiritual liberation.

Patanjali's worldview was dualist. In a dualist philosophy, the spiritual world and the material (physical) world are considered separate. In order to achieve liberation from suffering, the practitioner sought to escape the physical world and connect instead to the spiritual world. Practically speaking, this

For ease of communication, I will frequently refer to Yoga "texts." However, until the Middle Ages, most ideas and scriptures were memorized and transmitted orally rather than written down.

means that practitioners would renounce society, disregard the impulses of their bodies, and pursue and internally direct experience. Although this worldview may seem impractical (or even distasteful) to those of us who enjoy relationships, sensual delights, and the good company of others, *The Yoga Sutras* offers many profound insights on the nature of the mind and the human condition that remain universally relevant.

The Bhagavad Gita, translated as "The Lord's Song," is part of a vast epic called *The Mahabharata*, or "Great War." This sweeping story contains highly entertaining and dramatic tales of conflict, gods, romance, and magical creatures. In the Bhagavad Gita, we encounter Arjuna, a warrior on the brink of engaging in battle with the opposing side of his family. Although his cause for war is just, Arjuna is wracked with doubt and indecision as he considers the violence that will ensue.

Arjuna represents us. In our daily lives, we are also are often caught between a "rock and a hard place," where we don't know what to do. The Bhagavad Gita explores the essential conundrum: How can I be a yogi, when I sometimes have to do hurtful things? Is it possible to be a yogi and still participate in the world? The Bhagavad Gita provides an alternative to the traditionally ascetic practices of yoga, that promote renouncing society.

Fortunately, Arjuna has a trusted adviser on his side. Krishna is a god who appears as Arjuna's charioteer. Krishna represents the voice of our highest self, and inner wisdom. When Arjuna implores Krishna for help, Krishna reveals three yogic paths that will allow Arjuna to do his duty, or dharma, and uphold his spiritual integrity. These three paths are *jnana yoga*, *karma yoga*, and *bhakti yoga*, or the yoga of wisdom, action, and devotion, respectively. The Bhagavad Gita is a handbook for "living your yoga," and empowers practitioners to navigate the conflicts and drama of daily life with compassion, wisdom, and integrity.

52
CONTEMPLATIONS

1. WHO AM I?

Yogas Chitta Vritti Nirodhah

Since the dawn of consciousness, humans have been wrestling with the questions, Who am I? and How can I be happier?

For yogis, the answer begins with a fundamental mistake: we believe that we are what we think. In other words, we believe that thoughts such as I am a good person, I am a failure, I am a great mom, or I'm sad reflect our core identity. Let's look at this more closely.

The human mind is a spectacular engine of invention. Our capacity to connect disparate objects and ideas has spawned the invention of our greatest innovations, from early discoveries like metals, tools, and the wheel to more recent ones that have allowed us to traverse the continents, create global communication, and travel to the moon.

Although the mind is humankind's most powerful and precious tool, it comes with a dark side. The same power that propels innovation can also drive us to anxiety, depression, doubt, and despair. When we follow our thoughts into imagined shadow realities, we can become overwhelmed by negativity or fear.

To make it worse, we conflate our sense of self with this constantly changing and tumultuous landscape. When we think, I am good or I am bad we attach that label to our core identity. We assume that our sense of self is defined by what we think, feel, or do. When we think, I am a good worker, I am an accountant, I am a failure, or I am a success we believe that these labels define our core identify. But these labels are always changing.

"There is nothing either good or bad but thinking makes it so."

—William Shakespeare, from *Hamlet*

When I was younger, I moved from New York City to Vancouver, Canada, to embark upon a new life adventure with my fiancé. Before this great change, I had a comfortable and secure sense of self that was anchored to several identifiers: New Yorker, actor, loving girlfriend, American, strong woman.

Fast-forward a year: everything had fallen apart. My marriage had cracked open when my husband started drinking. I lived in a foreign country surrounded by strangers, and my career had disappeared. Suddenly, all of the happy identifiers I had previously enjoyed had been destroyed. My new labels were awful: expatriate, failed wife, obscure actor, enabler.

When we attach our sense of self with our changing and subjective experience, we set ourselves up for a wild roller-coaster ride of self-esteem.

Thousands of years ago, the yogis observed that our minds are always changing. Rather than attaching our sense of self to the constantly changing opinion of our minds, yogis offer a different point of view. They suggest attaching your sense of self to the part of you that is unwavering and consistent. This aspect of self is called *purusha*, which could be translated as your "soul," "higher consciousness," "presence," or "witness."

A Yoga text that was composed nearly 2,000 years ago, *The Yoga Sutras of Patanjali*, summarizes this understanding. The first few sutras capture the heart of the text. Loosely translated, they are:

▶ "Yoga is the restraint of the fluctuations of the mind stuff."

▶ "Then the seer (the self/witness/soul/consciousness) abides in (perceives) its own nature."

▶ "At other times, the Self appears to be the mind stuff."

In other words, when our minds are still, we perceive who we really are. When our minds aren't still, we mistake the content of our minds (the "mind stuff," like our thoughts and feelings) for our true selves.

Imagine that you are sitting by a lake. When the wind blows across the lake, the surface of the water is distorted. However, when the lake is calm, then the water can reflect the spaciousness of the sky. In the same way, when our minds (the lake) are disturbed by thoughts (the wind), then our true nature is obscured. But when our minds (the lake) are calm, they can reflect our true self or soul (the sky).

According to *The Yoga Sutras*, we are not our fluctuating thoughts or feelings; we are the presence, or purusha, that witnesses and observes our experiences. When we identify with purusha, rather than the content of our minds, we are in a state of yoga. When we are not present, our sense of self is misguidedly attached to our ever-changing thoughts and feelings.

Identifying with our minds can be called, "the great mistake." It is a classic case of mistaken identity in which we attach our sense of self to the wrong thing.

The yogis call this fundamental misperception *avidya*, which is Sanskrit for "non-seeing."

Thank goodness, it is surprisingly simple to correct this mistake.

By pausing and watching our thoughts, we can create space to question our habitual narratives. Simply put, we can choose to not believe everything we think. We can *watch* the story, rather than *be* the story.

One of my teachers explains this fundamental insight through the following story:

Imagine you are in a movie theater. You sit in your seat, the lights go down, and the movie comes on. Soon, you are so engrossed in the story that you forget you are watching a movie. When something exciting happens on the screen, you feel excitement. When something tragic happens, you feel sad. When there is happiness, you feel elated. When something scary happens, you feel afraid. But even though you are experiencing an emotional joyride, you have been safe in your movie seat the entire time.

We are like that moviegoer. We are immersed in the stories, emotions, relationships, and drama of a movie called, *My Life in A Human Body*. But while we may get caught up in the story, we are in reality quite safe as the unchanging witness watching the show.

When we can be less attached to the content of our stories—and more connected to the space of the witness—we can enjoy the wild ride of life without getting so frustrated by its changing and uncertain nature.

PRACTICE

▶ Take a comfortable seat.

▶ Close your eyes.

▶ Take a few deep, clearing breaths.

▶ Begin to notice your thoughts as they arise.

▶ Rather than follow your thoughts, instead allow yourself to watch them as they come and go.

▶ Enjoy the space between your thoughts.

▶ Sit in the seat of the watcher.

REFLECTION

▶ Throughout your day, pause to notice your thoughts. Are they true? What if they are not true?

▶ Who are you—your thoughts or the watcher?

2. LETTING GO OF BAGGAGE

Karma Yoga

Do you ever feel stuck in your stories, or in the "baggage" you carry with you from a previous experience?

For example, say that you were chased by a dog as a child. The outcome of that scary experience may be a fear of dogs, even though another dog may be quite friendly. If you have had your heart broken, you may become afraid of vulnerability and intimacy. Negative experiences usually create a reactive fear so that we avoid repeating the event. However, not all baggage is negative: a daily meditation practice may create a helpful mental routine for managing stress.

As a personal example, I was raised as a "nice" girl. I was taught to be polite, avoid conflict, and only speak when I had something nice to say. Although this training gave me a healthy respect for others' points of view, it also left me woefully ill equipped to wrestle with the interpersonal conflicts of my first marriage when my husband with alcoholism decided to start drinking again. To navigate my marriage, I had to recognize and question my habitual "nice girl" conditioning.

Ultimately, all of our experiences — good, bad, and ugly — leave an imprint that colors our perceptions of the world around us. According to the concept of karma, everything we do, think, feel, and say leaves an impression, or *samskara*. These imprints continue to accumulate throughout our lives, shaping the way we perceive and act. According to ancient yogis, the cycle of karma was a problem, as it doomed us to reincarnate into a continual cycle of suffering, or *samsara*. After all, if you keep creating karma when you're alive, then you'll just have to keep coming back to the world until you work it out. From a modern point of view, we might think of samskaras and karma as the habituation of neurological pathways. Neurons that "fire together, wire together." The more we practice certain behaviors or habits, the more conditioned we will become to repeat those same actions.

Although some of our habits may be useful (for example, a daily meditation practice that reduces stress), some may undermine our well-being (like a daily three-martini lunch). Changing our conditioning, particularly when it's become deeply engrained, requires the intention and willpower to change.

How can we navigate living a full, rich life and avoid the pitfalls of accumulating additional karma? The Bhagavad Gita provides a path. Composed around 500 BCE, the Bhagavad Gita was part of a great epic story called *The Mahabharata*. In this fantastical tale, the warrior Arjuna is given counsel by a god, Krishna.

Arjuna is in a bind similar to ours: How can we take action—particularly if it's going to create more conflict and karma—and also be a yogi? After all, living in the real world requires interacting with other people and taking action,

Karma: cycle of cause and effect; residue of the cycle of cause and effect

Samskara: impression, imprint

Samsara: the cycle of life and suffering

which naturally leads to karma and conditioning. So how can we be free?

Krishna outlined a revolutionary new type of yoga called karma yoga, or the yoga of action. According to Krishna, it is impossible to avoid action. As human beings living on the planet, we must breathe, eat, drink, walk, talk, and engage with the world. We cannot help but take action. Rather than avoid worldly interaction, Krishna suggested that attitude is everything. When we engage in action and are selfishly attached to the outcome, then we will create more karma. However, if we do our best in the moment and then surrender to the results of the actions, we can continue to be in the world karma free.

Consider this: How much of your thinking is caught up in what you did, what you should have done, what you could do, or your planning? Our mind's tendency to dwell on and rehash past regrets and future intentions keeps us from being fully in the present moment. But, if we could relinquish our attachment to outcomes, then we would be able to be more awake moment to moment.

Karma yoga invites us to be fully alive in the present moment by letting go of our relentless (and futile) attempts to control everything around us. Karma yoga asks us to be mindful of what we can actually control (our actions, right there and right now) and what we cannot (everything else).

> "Yoga is skill in action."
> —Bhagavad Gita

For example, I spent many years believing I was responsible for other people's reactions and feelings. Because of this mistaken viewpoint, I would bend over backward to avoid conflict, remain likeable, and keep the peace — which didn't always work. (If I actually had control over anyone else's feelings, I would be delighted to wave a wand and make everyone happy!)

By becoming clear about our own scope of responsibility, we are better able to take meaningful action, while recognizing the limits of our power.

REFLECTION

▶ How much of your thinking is devoted to replaying the past or imagining the future?

▶ What are you taking responsibility for now that is beyond your control?

▶ In what parts of your life can you take true responsibility for your own actions and agency?

▶ How does being in the present moment help you to make better choices?

3. LETTING GO OF FALSE IDENTITIES

Neti, Neti.

What makes you, you? Your clothes? Your job? Your body? The external trappings of your life can change. You can change clothes, jobs, your marital status, and where you live. But does this change who you really are?

Or, consider physical changes. Perhaps you dye your hair, grow older, sustain an injury, gain or lose weight, or change your gender. Do any of these changes alter who you really are?

To find what is eternal and unchanging, consider an ancient thought experiment called *neti, neti,* or "not this, not this." This exercise asks you to discard everything that is impermanent by saying, "I am not this." When you have discarded everything that you are not, you are left with (the perhaps indescribable) experience of what you are.

....

"Only to the extent that we expose ourselves over and over to annihilation can that which is indestructible in us be found."

—*When Things Fall Apart*, Pema Chodron

....

PRACTICE

Find a comfortable, easy seat. In this meditation, you will take time to consider some of the different elements in your life one by one. Consider if each element is a component of your core, unchanging identity. If it is not, then discard it by thinking, Not this.

Once you have completed a list of neti, neti, sit in the space of what remains.

Here are some examples of elements you might examine:

- ▶ I am not my clothes.
- ▶ I am not my family's behaviors.
- ▶ I am not my job.
- ▶ I am not my family.
- ▶ I am not my identity as a mother.
- ▶ I am not my face.
- ▶ I am not my weight.
- ▶ I am not my relationship.

- ▶ I am not my thoughts.
- ▶ I am not my feelings.
- ▶ I am not my anger.
- ▶ I am not my fear.
- ▶ I am not my ego.
- ▶ I am not my mistakes.
- ▶ I am not my addictions.
- ▶ I am not my habits.

REFLECTION

▶ When you find yourself feeling anxious or stressed, ask yourself, Where am I vesting my sense of self? What is false that I am protecting?

▶ In my confusion, what do I believe is *me* that is not me?

▶ Is the essential *me* — my true self — really at risk?

▶ When I pause, and take several deep breaths, is there really anything wrong in the present moment?

4. CONNECTING TO THE ABSOLUTE

Om

The word *om* is as old as the first Hindu texts, the Vedas, where it is used as an emphatic exclamation. By the time of *The Yoga Sutras*, Om was understood to represent *Isvara*, or "pure awareness." You can translate the term *Isvara* with a term that is personally resonant for you, such as universal consciousness, the absolute, the Lord, or cosmic intelligence.

In *The Yoga Sutras*, sutra 1.27–1.28, Patanjali reveals that Isvara is represented by the sound *om*, and that through the practice of repeating *om*, its essence may become clear.

In these sutras, Patanjali offers a potent and accessible tool for connecting to our highest selves: we can simply repeat the word *om*, and through this repetition, we will begin to naturally resonate with universal consciousness. In Yoga philosophy, Sanskrit words are not simply representations of objects; the sounds themselves embody the essence of what they describe. The repetition of words can therefore be extremely powerful.

Chanting *om* is like striking a tuning fork, in which we attune ourselves to a higher vibration. Not coincidentally, the sound of *om* is very similar to another sacred word, amen. The sound of both of these words invites us to resonate with something that is greater than ourselves.

The practice of Zen is forgetting the self in the act of uniting with something.

–Koun Yamada

PRACTICE

▶ Find a comfortable seat so that your spine is tall and easy.

▶ Take a few deep, slow breaths and focus on the sensations of your body.

▶ Quietly and slowly, repeat the mantra *om*, allowing yourself to sense the vibration of the sound.

▶ Repeat it 10 to 15 times.

▶ Rather than chanting *om* out loud, chant *om* silently to yourself about 10 times.

▶ Feel the internal vibration of the sound.

▶ Let the mantra go, and take a few deep breaths.

▶ Notice any shifts in your state of being.

5. CHANGING NEGATIVE THOUGHTS

Pratipaksha Bhavanam

We can be very hard on ourselves. The self-talk in our minds is often negative, critical, and driven by worry. When we start to believe in the spinning stories in our head, we can begin a spiral into anxiety or sadness.

In the *Yoga Sutras* 2.33, Patanjali says, *"Vitarka badhane pratipaksha bhavanam,"* which Swami Satchidananda translated as, "When disturbed by negative thoughts, opposite [positive] ones should be thought of."

How simple! How practical! And what a relief to recognize that humans have been struggling with bad thoughts for thousands of years.

Although the goal of yoga is ultimately to realize that we are presence (the inner witness, soul, or consciousness; in Sanskrit, *purusha*), it's useful to become friendly with our minds. Until we reach enlightenment and transcend our minds, we might as well cultivate a thought garden that is lush and nourishing rather than destructive. At the very least, considering ideas that challenge our mind's habitual judgments and criticisms will help create the space to recognize that the mind is subjective.

The judgment of the mind is often protective in nature. Over time, we have developed an "inner critic" voice to proactively protect us from failure, hurt, or vulnerability. However, left untended or unchallenged, we can start to believe the judgments in our heads are an accurate view of reality, rather than simply a protective mechanism.

Part of our personal growth is the practice of pausing so that we can question our conditioning, reevaluate our preexisting narratives, and see our situation from a more informed and compassionate perspective.

PRACTICE

Write out all the judgments that come into your mind. It may be useful to try this exercise for several days to keep a record of the many criticisms that arise and to notice any particular repetitions. The simple act of acknowledging and recording the voice of your inner critic will help you to create room from identifying with it.

For example, my own inner critic comments include:

▶ You're not fit.

▶ You're fat.

▶ You're not successful enough.

▶ You're lazy.

▶ You don't try hard enough.

▶ You're a crappy daughter.

▶ You're selfish.

For each judgment, write down a truthful antidote. If you have a hard time dislodging a criticism, then imagine the voice of an inner friend or cheerleader who can exuberantly defend you against these judgments.

Be energetic, enthusiastic, and unapologetic in your statements. The inner critic is an irrational tyrant who does not listen to reason; sometimes you just have to shout her down.

For my list, I might choose the following phrases as antidotes:

▶ I make healthy choices.

▶ I am beautiful at any size.

▶ I am successful.

▶ I work really hard.

▶ I am a loving and devoted daughter.

▶ Go away! (Or something stronger.)

Once you've written your antidotes, say them slowly and emphatically out loud in a strong, clear, and grounded voice.

Write out your favorite antidotes and post them somewhere that you can see them, or tuck them into your wallet.

REFLECTIONS

▶ Begin each day with a positive affirmation of your selfhood.

▶ Notice when the mind starts to travel on a familiar negative train, and use the emphatic statements of your "inner friend" to devalue and dismiss these judgments.

6. HOW TO RELATE TO HAPPY PEOPLE

Have you ever encountered someone who was happy...and it drove you crazy?

Although we may hope that we would be happy when someone else is joyful, sometimes that's not how it goes. Do any of these situations resonate with you?

▶ You've just entered a raffle for a free trip somewhere wonderful that you really, really, really want to win. But your friend wins the trip instead. You offer her congratulations, but are secretly jealous and sad that you didn't get the prize.

▶ You've been trying to get pregnant, but are having issues. Your friend shares the news that she is expecting. You want to be happy for her, but feel devastated.

▶ You have been struggling in your relationship. Your friend has just fallen madly in love and is waxing ecstatic about the wonder of romance. You roll your eyes and think, Yeah, just wait till it gets *real*.

▶ You're strapped for cash and have been working hard to make ends meet. Your sibling gets a promotion that comes with a spectacular raise.

If we aren't doing so well, or if someone seems to have something we want, then it can be challenging to feel friendly in the face of their happiness. Their happiness might seem to highlight our own sense of wanting.

For example, when I was an actress, competition for paying jobs was fierce. Often my friends and I would audition for the same role. Many times, they landed the job, and I didn't. Though I put on a cheerful face, my internal reaction to their good news was somewhere between self-flagellating despondency and bone-biting jealousy.

If I dug a little deeper, my reaction was a symptom of a much deeper problem: I was outsourcing the responsibility for my self-esteem to someone else. Rather than find a sense of wholeness and worthiness in myself, I was expecting that something outside of me—in this case, a job—would make me feel good about myself. In the acting business, I was usually giving a casting director—a perfect stranger—the keys to my self-esteem kingdom.

My self-criticism and sadness came from the misguided belief that my sense of worthiness depended on my professional success. Ironically, even if I *were* successful at an audition, my initial rush of confidence would dissipate with the next botched audition. I lacked stability in my own sense of self-worth.

Negatively reacting to another's happiness is usually a symptom of the great mistake. The great mistake occurs when we affix our sense of self and our worthiness to something outside of us. The material world, or *prakriti*, is constantly changing. After all, even mountains crumble eventually. When we rely on the external world—jobs, possessions, appearance, or reputation—to provide us with reassurance, we will ultimately be disappointed.

The yogis suggest that your true self, or purusha, is not subject to change, but is steady and eternal. You can connect to self by simply pausing, letting go of attachments to your thoughts, and connecting instead with the deep presence that is within you.

When you encounter happiness in others, practice (and it may indeed at first be a practice!) cultivating friendliness toward them and their situation. If you have negative feelings, trace them back to the root cause, and create space to connect to your own presence.

The more we practice cultivating friendliness toward those who are happy, the deeper our own sense of resilience, wholeness, and abundance will grow.

REFLECTION

- ▶ When have you struggled to delight in someone else's happiness?
- ▶ What lack in yourself were you imagining?
- ▶ Proactively practice cheerleading another in their happiness.
- ▶ Cultivate a small daily practice that helps you calm your mind and connect to the space of your presence.

7. HOW TO RELATE TO SAD PEOPLE

When someone is sad, how do you react?

- An acquaintance is devastated over an old breakup that was clearly for the best. Though you appreciate that she's sad, her moping is starting to get irritating.

- Your friend made a bundle on a hot stock tip, then lost it all. Though he's sad about the loss, you secretly feel relieved that you're not in his shoes.

- A former co-worker left your workplace with high hopes of branching out on her own. You'd always wanted to do the same, but were worried about the risk. When her business is struggling, you feel smug that you made the right choice.

Although we all wish we would react with a kind ear, sad people can bring impatience, frustration, discomfort, or even enjoyment to the surface.

Patanjali understood the human mind, and he knew that the majority of our internal drama can be triggered by other people. In sutra 1.33, he offers some practical advice for relating to others so that we have the best chance of retaining our equanimity—rather than being triggered and reactive. He advises that we cultivate *compassion* toward the unhappy. Interestingly, Patanjali is not recommending that we are compassionate because it will make us a good or moral person, but because compassion helps us to most easily retain our own peace of mind.

When we have an adverse reaction to someone's unhappiness, it is a sign that the other person's situation has triggered an attachment within us. Perhaps we feel uncomfortable because we relate too closely to their situation, or we might feel relieved that we have escaped their unfortunate fate. When we do not react with compassion, it's a sign to dig deeper in ourselves and notice what is really going on.

One of my friends was involved in a very intense relationship with her girlfriend. They would continually break up, then get back together, only to break up again. My friend was often perpetually sad that they couldn't resolve their differences and would bemoan their relationship's on-and-off-again status. Rather than feeling compassion for her, I instead felt irritated and frustrated. I wanted to give her a good smack on the side of the head and say, "Snap out of it, already!"

Digging a little deeper into my reaction, I realized that I felt triggered because my friend was repeating the exact same behavior I had exhibited in a previous relationship of my own. Her situation reminded me all too clearly of how confused and sad I had felt in similar circumstances and I didn't like being reminded of my behavior.

Cultivating a true attitude of compassion toward the unhappy is not simply about putting on a sympathetic face and saying the right words. The real work is to recognize when there is an obstacle to our natural empathy, and to root out what has triggered our reaction. In this way, we can clear away the obstacles to our own goodwill, so that our compassion may flow easily and naturally. From an authentic open heart, we can then hold space that is genuine, loving, and supportive for others.

8. HOW TO RELATE TO VIRTUOUS PEOPLE

Have you ever seen a movie that involved police corruption? Usually, there's a cop on the take who is trying to convince his new and idealistic partner that it's okay to accept "protection money." The new partner resists crossing the line, much to the consternation and anger of the corrupt officer. Drama ensues!

In this movie plot, the corrupt police officer is not very happy with the "virtuosity" of his partner.

Perhaps you can relate to some of these other ways that we may react to people who are virtuous:

▶ Your friend raves about her new green-smoothie health food kick, and you've just chowed down your second doughnut. Rather than congratulating your friend on her virtuousness, you poke despondently at your belly and lament your lack of discipline.

▶ You desperately need to vent about your irritating coworker, and your friend gently reminds you that she doesn't like to participate in gossip. You feel irritated that she is so judgmental.

▶ You're finally out for a fun night on the town, and suggest that everyone gets a second round of drinks. Your friend passes, saying that she wants to stay clearheaded and doesn't like to drink too much. You feel deflated and annoyed.

According to sutra 1.33, Patanjali advises us to "delight in the virtuous."

A virtuous person could be described as someone who is upholding the elevation of their own values at the expense of personal comfort. Upholding values could include donating time to a good cause, making healthy food choices, or using money conscientiously. On a grander scale, upholding one's values could involve standing up to tyranny or exposing corruption at personal expense.

Although it seems that we should naturally admire the virtuous, virtuosity can be irritating when it exposes our own *lack* of virtuosity.

For example, let's say that you are out with a friend, and you want to order dessert. "Want to split something?" you say, hoping your companion will indulge with you. She demurs, "No, I'm avoiding sugar these days." You may feel disappointed and even irritated that your friend won't get off her high horse and have a little fun.

In this moment, your friend's refusal to join you in dessert exposes your own internal conflict. If you felt 100 percent okay about eating dessert, you would cheerfully order the double chocolate fudge cake. Instead, her refusal sparks your own internal conflict between the sensual enjoyment of eating something delicious, and supporting the longevity of your own health. If she had joined you in dessert, you could have swept your internal conflict under the rug. But her refusal puts you in the uncomfortable position of having to consciously acknowledge your own choice.

When we don't experience an instinctive "delight" in the virtuous, it's a sign that we are experiencing an internal conflict between what we want to do — and what we believe we *should* do. Our values are in conflict, and we don't like the way it feels. In response, we may feel defensive, exposed, or defiant.

From an objective point of view, virtuous actions should instill admiration. After all, the world is a better place when humans are willing to be uncomfortable in order to do the right thing.

When someone else's virtuosity triggers us it is a sign that we need to do some internal work on our own values. We can either buck up and practice doing the "hard thing," or we can practice self-acceptance and embrace that we are the kind of person that occasionally just loves to eat cake. In either scenario, the responsibility for self-consciousness is ours.

REFLECTION

▶ As you move through your day, notice the choices that you are making. What values are you upholding?

▶ When you are indecisive, which values are in conflict?

▶ Consider someone you admire. Which values are they upholding that you wish to develop in yourself?

9. HOW TO RELATE TO WICKED PEOPLE

Swami Satchidananda translates sutra 1.33 as: "By cultivating attitudes of friendliness toward the happy, compassion for the unhappy, delight in the virtuous, and disregard toward the wicked, the mind-stuff retains its undisturbed calmness."

Consider the following scenarios:

► Your coworker is clearly slacking on work and not pulling his own weight, and it's driving you crazy! Every time you see him getting coffee or chatting on the phone, you want to throw your laptop at him.

► You see a bully on a playground, picking on a smaller kid, and want to give her a dose of her own medicine.

► The news is running story after story about large companies that are cheating on regulations and dumping illegal pollutants into the oceans. You feel despair.

How do we respond when faced with wickedness? When we cannot change the situation, disregarding the wicked can be useful for our own peace of mind.

For example:

► You refrain from getting into a futile debate with someone you consider to have damaging political views.

▶ You have no control to change a situation or something bad that has happened in the past.

If you are interested in justice, then Patanjali's advice to "disregard" the wicked may seem like a hard pill to swallow. Patanjali wasn't interested in saving the world or punishing the unjust; his priority was to help you retain the calmness of your mind.

However, although we want to avoid ruminating over someone else's wickedness, this does not mean that we cannot take action to rectify a wrong. In sutra 1.33, Patanjali advises you to have "compassion for the unhappy" and to "delight in the virtuous."

When you see a bully picking on someone at the playground, "disregarding the wicked" may not be as important as having "compassion for the unhappy" or "delighting in the virtue" of fairness. Out of compassion for the bully's victim, you may choose to take action.

Whether or not we act, Patanjali would advise us to notice the state of our mind. Are we able to let the remembrance of these wicked acts go, or do we continue to give them a life of their own within our heads?

In one story, an old monk and a young monk walk down to the river. A beautiful woman is trapped on this side of the river. The old monk carries her across the river and she goes on her way. After a couple more miles of walking, the younger monk finally bursts out, "We have taken a vow of celibacy. How could you carry that woman across the river?" The old monk looks surprised and says, "My dear boy, I left her there. Why are you still carrying her?"

REFLECTION

When you feel upset by someone else's unscrupulous acts, consider:

▶ Do you have the power to change circumstances for the better?

▶ Will taking action ease the rumination of your mind?

▶ If not, what do you gain by continuing to hold on to it?

10. WHY AM I HERE?

Dharma

Many yoga traditions would propose that your goal in this incarnation is to recover your connection with your truest nature, and to yoke your identification to your true self. Through the practice of yoga and meditation, you can begin the process of self-realization, and recognize that your core identity is not attached to your thoughts and feelings, but is uncovered when you connect to your internal witness, or presence. You experience yoga (union) when you are properly connected to this deep awareness that lies within.

This is the soul's purpose, to remember its personal and eternal connection to the divine. From a yogic perspective, you don't have to work to create the connection; it's who you fundamentally are. The work is to remove the obstacles that stand in the way of this realization.

Although remembering our intrinsic divinity is certainly nice, we may also be interested in worldly work. According to the Bhagavad Gita, our dharma or duty, is our worldly purpose. We are instructed that it is better to do our own dharma, no matter how humble, than to do someone else's, no matter how exalted.

Tat tvam asi: thou art that. You are what you are seeking.

It is important to ask "What does life want of me?" We are usually consumed with trying to get something from life; how refreshing and what a relief to think instead of what we are here to provide!

Sometimes we can become afraid if we don't connect to a grand purpose in our life. I should know what my purpose is or what I need to do, we may worry. Instead, ask, "What is this present moment asking of me?" Start moment to moment. This moment may be asking you to read this book, rest your body, be a compassionate ear for a friend, earn a living, support your children, or take care of your body. Each moment will bring an opportunity to explore your own purpose—and how you can live your yoga.

> "Ultimately, man should not ask what the meaning of his life is, but rather must recognize that it is he who is asked. In a word, each man is questioned by life; and he can only answer to life by *answering for* his own life; to life he can only respond by being responsible."
>
> —Viktor E. Frankl, *Man's Search for Meaning*

Your dharma can change over the course of your life. At one point you may be dedicated to your studentship, and at another time it may be your highest value to be good mother. By revisiting What does life want from me?, we can stay open to fresh impulses and information.

As another point of view, according to bhakti yoga (yoga of devotion), the greatest purpose we have is to love. Every act is performed as an expression of devotion and reverence. No matter what worldly work we undertake, we can give our actions meaning by infusing them with our love. When in doubt, add love to your actions and you will never go wrong.

REFLECTION

▶ What is asking from me?

▶ In the past, have I had moments in which I have been clear on my purpose? What gave me that feeling of clarity?

▶ Beneath the mind's voices of fear, criticism, or judgment, is there something that my soul is calling me to do?

▶ What types of activities bring me joy?

11. INTENSITY

Tapas

Throughout yoga history, fire has been used for purification and transformation. In the time of the Vedas, priests performed ritual sacrifices and used smoke to send sacrifices to the gods. Later, yogis engaged in austerities (purification practices) such as fasting and abstinence, and used the "fire" of their discipline to harness their minds. During the time of *The Yoga Sutras*, Patanjali named fire as an essential component of a yogi's practice. Today, we use the intensity of the physical practice to make our bodies stronger and help focus our minds.

Tapas literally means "heat," and can be translated as, "the willingness to endure intensity for the sake of transformation." Yogis recognized that change involves discomfort; we need some fire to hold to a new course of action rather than slide into the comfort of a familiar habit.

Humans are wired to seek the path of least resistance. However, the path of least resistance often won't get us what we really want. To our goals—be they worldly or spiritual—we need some grit. Intensity can take many forms, and arises most often when we are confronted with a challenge or change. Staying present when comfortable routines are tested requires fortitude.

For example, I can feel a good deal of intensity if I wake up in the morning and find out that I'm out of coffee, challenging my creature comforts. I also experience the heat of tapas when my yoga teacher asks me to hold plank pose longer than I may like. Though I may start to shake, I can recognize the value in confronting my own perceived limitations. Psychologically, I experienced a great deal of personal intensity when my engrained identify as a "nice girl" who avoided conflict began to shift. I had to learn to unravel years of conditioning to find a voice and speak up for myself in a healthy way.

It's important to note that tapas is intensity *for the sake of transformation*. We aren't engaging in discomfort pointlessly, or simply to develop power. We challenge ourselves because we wish to uphold a higher value beyond our personal comfort. By mindfully engaging in tapas, we can generate the necessary fire to clear old habits, make changes, and consciously manifest our will in the world.

REFLECTION

Recall a time of great intensity:

▶ How did intensity serve you?

▶ What did you learn?

▶ Would the learning have been possible without the intensity?

As you encounter intensity, ask:

▶ Is this intensity for a higher purpose?

▶ What value am I upholding by challenging myself?

12. SEXUALITY

Brahmacharya

For much of its history, Yoga philosophy advised practitioners to be celibate. After all, because the goal of yoga is to create equanimity in the mind, it made sense to advocate practices that avoided riling us up. You only have to think back to your big first crush to remember how much sexual attraction can create a thought tornado! To avoid this tumult, yogis practiced *brahmacharya*, or abstinence. After all, if temptation is off the table, then the mind may have a better chance of staying calm.

Early yogis were not impressed with the world or their bodies in general. They believed that the material/ physical world (prakriti) and the spiritual world (purusha) were separate. Connecting to one's spiritual nature meant focusing on their internal experiences and avoiding distractions of the body, including pleasure, food, alcohol, and sex.

With the emergence of tantric philosophy around the sixth century, a more positive attitude toward the world—and body—emerged. According to tantric philosophy, the material world is the unfolding expression of universal consciousness.

Let's explore what that means.

First, what is universal consciousness? Universal consciousness is divine intelligence and awareness. You might also call it God, soul, collective consciousness, cosmos, or universal love. The tantric yogis called it *shiva*. At an individual level, it's known as purusha.

On the other hand, there is the energy of manifestation called *shakti*. Ultimately, shakti is responsible for the expression of prakriti, which is composed of the five elements, or *mahabhutas*: earth, air, water, fire, ether. Everything in the physical world is subject to the *gunas*, or forces of nature. Unlike the steadiness of shiva, shakti is in constant flux. Everything that is part of shakti has a cycle: arising, sustaining, dissolving, then arising again. In tantric philosophy, shakti and shiva are two sides of the same coin. If you think of a candle, shakti is the flame, and shiva is the light. You can't have one without the other.

Here is another way to think of it from the point of view of physics:

If you imagine the universe before the big bang, all of space, time, energy, consciousness, and matter was condensed into one impossible singularity. This singularity is expressive of the fundamental unity of shiva-shakti. Once the big bang occurred, this singularity expanded into a multiplicity of elements, including space, time, and matter. The consciousness and intelligence of the universe would be shiva, but the matter and energy within it are shakti. However, traced back to their source—and from the highest perspective—they are one.

So, what does all this mean for sexuality?

Before tantra, the material world—shakti—was generally regarded as an impediment to the spiritual practice. Ascetic yogis would avoid the sensual pleasures of the world entirely and focus exclusively on their connection with the spiritual. However, with this new perspective, the material world was regarded as an essential aspect of divine consciousness. The body and its senses could actually be used as a vehicle for connection with the divine.

Tantra opened the door for the inclusion of sensory and body-based meditation practices. The senses were regarded as *devis*, or goddesses, who needed to be nourished. More subtle body practices involving sound and visualizations were developed. Over time, this body-centric perspective led to the postural yoga practice called hatha yoga (from which the modern style of yoga called "hatha" took its name).

The tantric and hatha yogis were very mindful of the role that sexual energy played in the cultivation of our life essence, or *ojas*. They developed practices to conserve, build, and harness this bodily energy, including increasing sexual energy without orgasm.

Given our modern culture, brahmacharya does not have to be interpreted as a prescription for chastity. However, it is an invitation to be aware of the power of our own sexuality and to use it wisely. In our culture, sexuality has been commodified and used as a marketing tool to sell everything from beer to cars. Casual sex has been glorified, and the misuse of sexual energy and power has been exposed in almost every aspect of contemporary culture, including yoga.

Brahmacharya invites us to explore our personal relationship with this powerful part of our nature, so that we can be aware of its potential and use it with awareness.

Consider the following:

▶ Do your sexual relationships serve you (this includes your sexual relationship with yourself)?

▶ Are you depleted or nourished in your relationship to your sexual energy?

▶ If you have a partner(s), how are they served by the relationship?

More broadly, brahmacharya invites you to investigate how you are replenishing, conserving, and using your vital energy in all areas of your life.

REFLECTION

▶ What activities do you find energetically depleting?

▶ What activities do you find nourishing?

▶ On the whole, how is your energy?

▶ What self-care practices can you use to refill your own energetic well?

13. PLEASURE

Raga

The Chariot Story (adapted from the Katha Upanishad)

Once upon a time, there was a chariot being pulled by five horses named Smell, Sight, Hearing, Taste, and Touch. Excited by everything around them, those horses ran after whatever new and delicious experience came across their path.

Carrots! Hay! The wind!

The horses' desire to pursue pleasure didn't make them bad horses; they were simply following the call of their nature.

There was a charioteer at the reins, named the mind. If the charioteer wasn't paying proper attention, the horses would race in every direction. But when the charioteer was present, the horses could be steered with intention.

However, the chariot only really got where it was supposed to go when the charioteer listened to the chariot's passenger, the soul. When the mind listened to the soul, then the chariot found its way to the proper destination.

We are wired for pleasure. In Sanskrit, pleasure is called *raga*. It is quite natural that our senses will pull us toward objects that bring pleasure. In sutra 2.7, Patanjali writes, "Attachment is a residue of a pleasant experience." From a neurological point of view, we seek to repeat experiences that fire up our brain's pleasure center.

However, our senses and our lower mind, *manas*, don't have consciousness. They are part of the "mind layer" of our experience *(manomaya kosha)* and lack discrimination and discernment. Left to pursue their own desires, our senses will indulge again and again in what brings them pleasure, whether it's wine, sugar, sex, or chocolate.

We may also use pleasure inappropriately, in order to cover up feelings of unworthiness, anxiety, sadness, or wanting. After all, it can seem far easier to reach for the glass of wine or tub of ice cream than to sit in our uncomfortable feelings.

Manas: mind

Manomaya kosha: the mind layer

"[Manomaya kosha is] where the incessant thoughts of human life occur."

—B.K.S. Iyengar, *Light on Life*

As the chariot story tells us, only when our highest self (our soul, purusha, self, witness) directs the horses do we truly move in the direction that serves our highest good.

Pleasure has always been a thorny issue for humankind. Early yogis chose to avoid the temptations of pleasure entirely, choosing instead to practice celibacy, fasting, and cleansing to avoid the distraction of pleasure. Many spiritual traditions have followed (and continue to follow) a similar path, preaching celibacy and advocating for the control or even suppression of the body.

The development of tantric yoga heralded a worldview that considered our bodies, our senses, and the world as the living fabric of the divine. Pleasure, at last, had a place in the spiritual human experience. Rather than be avoided and shunned, pleasure was recognized as an essential and valuable component of human experience.

> "We must increase our tolerance for pleasure."
>
> —Gil Hedley, PhD

However, tantric yogis also recognized that engaging in pleasure required a more sophisticated level of consciousness: the greater the pleasure, the more mindful we need to be. Creating a relationship with pleasure is far more challenging in some ways than avoiding it entirely. Perhaps you've experienced this for yourself: it can be easier to eliminate a pleasurable item entirely than to try to enjoy something in moderation.

Once we start to enjoy something—sugar, alcohol, cigarettes, sex, spending money, watching TV, gambling, engaging in social media—it can be hard for us to stop. Some pleasures are hard to control.

As yogis, our work is to become aware of our relationship to pleasure so that we may enjoy sensual delights fully and with integrity. Pleasure, sensuality, and beauty are birthrights of our human experience. Experiencing the warmth of sunshine, taking a deep breath, touching the softness of cashmere, and tasting delicious food are all gifts of our embodiment. Through mindfulness, we can increase our awareness of the pleasures in the present moment, and create a positive relationship with our sensual side.

PRACTICE

Eat one thing slowly:

▶ Choose a small amount of food that you really love. It could be something like a piece of chocolate, a raisin, a small piece of pizza, a strawberry. (preferably something that won't melt).

▶ Pause.

▶ Take in the food first with all of your senses except taste.

▶ After you have thoroughly explored it with your other senses, then very slowly, take a small bite.

▶ Roll it in your mouth to explore its texture, its different flavors.

▶ Give yourself over to the pleasure of the experience.

▶ Chew it many times.

▶ Slowly, small bite by small bite, begin to eat the food.

When you are finished, reflect:

▶ How was that experience different from your habitual approach to this food?

▶ How could this inform a new relationship to pleasure?

REFLECTION

- ▶ What is my current relationship to pleasure?
- ▶ Where can I make the time to experience pleasure in its fullest spectrum?
- ▶ Where and why do I not permit myself to experience pleasure?
- ▶ Where and why do I lose control and overindulge?
- ▶ When do I use pleasure to cover up uncomfortable feelings?
- ▶ Are there beliefs around pleasure I could revisit?

14. CONFLICT

Jnana Yoga

How can we be yogis, and engage in conflict? For most of us, the idea of engaging in violence and practicing yoga seem diametrically opposed. How can we resolve this seeming contradiction?

This paradox was one of the core issues explored in the great yogic text, the Bhagavad Gita. In the Gita, the warrior Arjuna is about to begin a great battle with his family. Although Arjuna is in the right, he can't fathom how killing his own family could possibly lead to any good. He throws down his weapons in despair and will not fight.

Like us, Arjuna is stuck. He realizes that he should take action, and yet can't abide the consequences that his actions will cause. We all know what it's like to be stuck between a rock and a hard place.

Soon after I was married, my spouse became despondent because his mother had died and he began drinking. Unfortunately, he also suffered from alcoholism. As time went on, he became emotionally abusive and I became increasingly enabling and withdrawn. I felt trapped between my commitment as a wife and friend and my growing unhappiness. I didn't know what to do.

Although the "right choice" in this scenario may seem more clear to me now, in the moment I felt consumed by doubt and indecision.

You have certainly experienced your own "rock and a hard place" moment, perhaps at work, with kids, with family, or in romantic relationships. As yogis who live in the world (rather than retreating to a cave for meditation), we will naturally be embroiled in the drama and chaos of daily life and conflict. So how do we choose what to do?

In the Bhagavad Gita, Arjuna is being advised by his charioteer, Krishna, who also (fortunately!) happens to be a god. Krishna represents the voice of our highest inner wisdom, or *buddhi*.

To help Arjuna navigate his situation, Krishna offers him three paths to insight: jnana yoga, karma yoga, and bhakti yoga. Although these three forms of yoga are slightly different, they are united by one guiding principle: *View the situation from the highest perspective*.

When we are debating a choice in our minds, we are always going to be stuck in competing stories. Should I do this? Should I do that? Our minds can justify any decision or point of view, so we will be left in confusion. Listening to just our feelings can provide some information, though fear or discomfort can distort them. Instead of making a decision based on thoughts and feelings, we must attune to the voice of our highest self, and be guided by our highest values.

In jnana yoga, the yoga of wisdom, we practice pausing so that we can step out of the tumult of thoughts and feelings, and return to a deeper, guiding sense of presence.

We can do this through a simple process:

▶ Pause.

- Take a few deep, slow breaths.
- Begin to observe your thoughts and feelings.
- Create space for all your thoughts and feelings to arise, be felt, and then dissipate or change.
- Begin to be the witness of what is arising for you.
- Be the space beyond the thoughts, rather than the thoughts.
- Be the space beyond the feelings, rather than the feelings.
- Stand in the space of the witness, rather than the story.

From this higher perspective, we can recognize our own intrinsic wholeness and a consistent sense of deep presence. When we are connected to self, we remember that we are fundamentally safe and are not as attached to things turning out a certain way. We know that we are okay—and we know that (in the case of relationship) the other will also be okay. Much of the drama that happens in our heads is because we have misguided attachment to a circumstances that must change. From this place, we can more easily see the highest path forward.

In the Bhagavad Gita, Arjuna eventually goes into battle. However, he is not going into battle for the sake of his ego, for material gain, or because he is emotionally reactive. He engages in battle because it is the highest action he can take to support justice and uphold his values.

Like Arjuna, when we feel we must do battle, our first job is to pause, connect more deeply with ourselves, and become clear on our highest values. We cannot avoid conflict, but we can do our best to make sure that we are entering the battlefield for the best reasons.

REFLECTION

Reflect upon and observe your own relationship to conflict:

▶ What is my relationship to conflict?

▶ Do I engage in battle for petty, selfish, or ego-centered reasons? If so, why? What do I perceive that I will gain? Is it true?

▶ Do I shrink from conflict, even when for the highest good? If so, why? What do I perceive that I will gain? Is it true?

▶ How can I support myself to be a spiritual warrior?

15. CONNECTION AND LOVE

Bhakti Yoga

Have you ever noticed that when you feel happy, safe, and full of love, you are naturally more compassionate, generous, energetic, and kind to others?

The nature of the world is love. One of the forms of yoga that Krishna imparted in the Bhagavad Gita, bhakti yoga, is the yoga of devotion, in which practitioners love their way into their highest self.

Try this:

▶ Pause and take a comfortable set.

▶ Close your eyes and take a few slow, deep breaths.

▶ Give yourself the space of a minute or so to notice the thoughts and feelings that arise.

▶ After a minute, bring to mind the face of someone you love unconditionally. This could be a person (living or deceased), but could also be a beloved pet.

▶ See their face, study their aspect, and allow the feelings you have for this creature to arise within you.

▶ After a minute or so, allow your visualization of the beloved to be released.

▶ Notice how you feel now. What has changed?

When we are in contact with a personal beloved (this doesn't need to be romantic love), we are connected with the essence of our own human heart. We experience softness, kindness, vulnerability, and we can more easily experience the good in others.

We can then extend this feeling of beneficence and goodwill beyond our personal beloved and begin to experience the essence and interconnectedness of the greater world. Not only our human communities, but we can also feel the divine interconnection of nature and all creatures everywhere.

We can also start with an appreciation for the magnificence of the divine, and allow that love to infuse the smallest details of our daily lives. Every act becomes an expression of devotion, reverence, and love. To the bhakti yogi, everything is an expression of the divine.

From the perspective of bhakti yogis, everything is connected. When we see the interconnectedness of all things, we can begin to love others as we love ourselves. And if we struggle with self-love, our increasing ability to see the beauty in others will allow us—as a reflection—to see the magnificence in ourselves.

"May all beings everywhere be happy and free."

Lokah Samastah Sukhino Bhavantu

—Sanskrit mantra

PRACTICE

- ▶ Take a comfortable seat.

- ▶ Take a few deep breaths and close your eyes.

- ▶ Focus on your breath.

- ▶ Bring to mind the face of someone you love. Take a few moments to imagine their details or how they make you feel.

- ▶ Think, Just like me, you want to be happy. Repeat this until you feel it.

- ▶ Bring to mind the face of someone you are neutral about. Take a few moments to imagine their details or how they make you feel.

- ▶ Think, Just like me, you want to be happy. Repeat this until you feel it.

- ▶ Bring to mind the face of someone with whom you may have challenges. Take a few moments to imagine their details or how they make you feel.

- ▶ Think, Just like me, you want to be happy. Repeat this until you feel it.

- ▶ Imagine that you could encompass the whole world in your meditation: Just like me, you want to be happy.

- ▶ When you are ready, take a few deep breaths and experience what you feel.

REFLECTION

▶ What is my relationship to self-love?

▶ What are the obstacles to loving myself, or to loving others?

▶ Where (or for whom) do I feel unconditional love and devotion?

▶ How can I practice experiencing this love so that I can love others and myself more freely and with wonderful abandon?

16. NONVIOLENCE, COMPASSION

Ahimsa

In *The Yoga Sutras*, Patanjali shares an eight-limbed path called ashtanga yoga, which details eight components of the spiritual life. You can imagine these eight limbs as the roots of a tree, each one nourishing and sustaining the whole.

The first limb is called the *yamas*, which can be translated as "external disciplines." There are five yamas, each of which directs us in how to interact with the external world with integrity.

The first yama is *ahimsa*, which can be translated as "nonviolence." In Chip Hartranft's translation of sutra 2.35, Patanjali shares that "Being firmly grounded in nonviolence creates an atmosphere in which others can let go of their hostility."

Have you ever noticed that it "takes two to tango" where conflict is concerned? When we are able to relate to others from a space of compassion, rather than opposition, we can usually navigate our relationships with more grace.

Our anger usually emerges when the way the world is and the way we want the world to be are not aligned. We feel that the power of our anger (frustration, irritation, or rage) will somehow change the world more to our liking.

Although such emotions are natural, they usually result from a fundamental confusion: we have mistakenly vested our sense of self with the constantly changing world, rather than identifying with our true nature. In this confusion, we believe that our sense of safety and wholeness is associated with something outside of ourselves. For example, we identify strongly with our jobs, or our identity as a good worker or good dad. When these identities and stories are threatened, we rear up and fight back. Anger is always protective in nature, and emerges when we want to put the world back to rights.

However, if we were truly grounded and settled within ourselves, we would have no need to fight for anyone else's good opinion. Our own sense of wholeness would require no external affirmation or defense.

However, learning to identify with our core self — rather than the stories in our minds — takes practice. Practice, or *abhyasa*, is a continual, resilient, and loving intent to recognize that our true identity is the presence that lies beyond our thoughts and feelings, beyond our stories and reactions.

Rather than think about yamas — and ahimsa — as ethical guidelines to follow, you can instead think of them as signposts that you are on the right path. When we are correctly identified with our true nature (our presence, rather than the stories in our minds), we are less likely to get angry over something not working out the way we want.

We don't need to *try* to be non-violent; as we practice our yoga, we will become naturally more compassionate because the need to defend our egos will gradually start to drop away.

REFLECTION

▶ When do you express violence toward yourself? This can take the form of nonacceptance, judgment, or criticism.

▶ When you are angry, consider what you are trying to protect. Does it really need protecting?

17. TRUTHFULNESS

Satya

Have you ever had to keep a secret?

In one of my relationships, I wanted children, and my partner did not. Every time we spoke of the issue, we would find ourselves at a stalemate. Rather than face the huge elephant in the room and make the necessary changes, we instead began to live inside a bubble of denial and deceit.

The relationship was unsustainable. Every moment between us was weighed down by the heaviness of what was unspoken and we both grew increasingly unhappy. Through admitting the truth was very painful, it ultimately brought us clarity and peace.

> "The truth will set you free."
> —John 8:32

In *The Yoga Sutras*, the first limb of an eight-limbed path of yoga is called the *yamas*, which can be translated as "external disciplines." There are five yamas; the first yama is ahimsa, or non-violence, and the second yama is *satya*, or truthfulness. Patanjali writes in sutra 2.36, "For those grounded in truthfulness, every action and its consequences are imbued with truth" (translation, Chip Hartranft).

When we lie, our minds become anxious and divided. The lie demands that we remember what we have said, and give energy to maintaining its story. It can be hard for us to remain present and open when we have to devote energy to maintaining a fiction.

When we are truthful, we can more easily remain steady and clear. In our truthfulness, we empower others around us to live their truth as well.

Have you ever noticed that sometimes a hard conversation is worse to anticipate than to actually have? Dishonesty undermines authentic connection. When we are honest — even when it's hard — true connection is possible. Even when the truth leads to an honest willingness to "agree to disagree" (as can happen in my family's political conversations), truthfulness allows us to become more intimate and loving with others because we come out of hiding.

But if telling the truth is such a good idea, then why do we lie?

When I was a little girl, I used to respond to new information by pretending I already knew it. "I know," I'd reply, to any new tidbit. Being a little girl, I didn't understand a lot, so I was saying, "I know," a lot! My dad finally took my aside, and said, "You don't have to say that you know. It's okay not to know."

I remember feeling caught off guard. I had been saying, "I know," because I thought that knowing stuff would make me look good. Not knowing felt vulnerable and scary. While I could pretend that lying to save face was simply a little girl's folly, fast-forward 40 years and I'm still tempted to avoid admitting I don't know things.

One of my acquaintances cheated on his wife for eight years. Rather than have an honest conversation about his unhappiness, he thought it was kinder to leave her in the dark. She'd be so hurt, he justified to himself, and my kids would be devastated. Although both of these things may have been true, his primary motivation for lying was to protect himself from dealing with their disappointment. He didn't want to face the consequences of speaking his truth, and so he chose to lie for almost a decade.

Lying isn't only about what you say; it can also be about what you don't say.

For example, it's a common practice to "ghost" someone in the dating world, where one party disappears without further communication. She'll get it eventually, the ghoster may think, as he deletes his date's text message. But in the meantime, the other person has been left in the dark, wasting time thinking that the relationship may go somewhere. Rather than share an honest and immediate (if uncomfortable) accounting of their feelings, ghosters leave dates to linger in uncertainty for days.

We often tell ourselves that we are lying to protect someone else. But in reality, we almost always lie to protect ourselves. Here's the tricky part: embracing truthfulness isn't as simple as blurting out everything we're feeling and thinking.

As the yamas suggest, honesty rests in the gracious arms of compassion. Without compassion, blunt honesty can be needlessly hurtful and self-serving. To live satya in our lives, we must pause to consider if our expression of the truth is serving the greatest good. Is it needed? Is it helpful? When the truth can't help, then silence may be the most compassionate course. But if the truth will honor the personhood of someone else, then it may be our responsibility to share it.

One of the hardest moments of my life was telling my ex-husband that I wasn't in love with him anymore. I did not share this information to be cruel; I shared it with him so that he could move on in his own best interests and find a new relationship that would be fulfilling. I said it so that we would both be free.

Rather than think about yamas—and satya—as ethical rules, you can also think of them as signposts that you are on the right path. When we are correctly identified with our true nature (our Presence, rather than the stories in our minds), we are less likely to feel the need to protect our ego by creating fabrications or distorting the truth.

REFLECTION

▶ What is your relationship to speaking your truth?

▶ What gets in the way of you communicating honestly?

▶ Are there areas in your life in which you would like to create more honesty and truthfulness?

18. WHY WE FORGET

The Five Acts

You go to yoga class, experience a profound sense of peace and a loving appreciation for everyone around you. Then on the way home, someone cuts you off in traffic. "You idiot!" you holler. And just like that, divine connection goes *poof*.

If our true nature is to be one with the universe, then why do we keep forgetting ourselves so often?

According to tantric text, *The Heart of Recognition*, written by Rajanaka Kshemaraja around 1000 CE, the Divine is constantly performing five acts. And because we are part of the divine fabric, we are also constantly performing these five acts:

▶ The first act, *srsti*, is the act of creation. Through this act, the divine manifests into form. This could be the manifestation of anything: thought, a flower, or a human.

▶ The second act, *sthiti*, is stasis. Through this act, something holds its form.

▶ The third act, *samhara*, is reabsorption. Through this act, what has been in form is reabsorbed back into consciousness.

▶ The fourth act, *tirodhana*, is concealment. Through this act, the divine conceals its nature, or its qualities.

▶ The final and fifth act is *anugraha*, or revelation, through which the divine is revealed.

Tirodhana helps explain why we are constantly forgetting our true nature. Concealment is an essential aspect in the play of the divine. This act explains why we may experience glimpses of grace *(anugraha)*, only to find our understanding veiled once again.

The five acts are enormously comforting. It's as if the text lovingly puts a hand on our shoulder and whispers, "It's okay to forget, that's part of your journey, too."

REFLECTION

▶ What does it mean for you if the third act, samhara, does not mean "ending" or "death," but "reabsorption"?

▶ What is your typical reaction to your own forgetting?

▶ What activities allow you to reconnect with the fifth act, revelation?

19. STICKINESS

Asteya | Aparigraha

Have you ever gotten exactly what you wanted, only to be quickly dissatisfied and then have a hard time letting it go again? Our tendency to want something—then hold it tightly to us—is very human.

As a tangible example, my mom and dad have very different ideas about holding on to material possessions. My dad rolls his eyes at the accumulation of stuff in the garage, while my mother gasps in outrage. "You can't get rid of that," she'd say. "Rachel wore that dress when she was seven at her second-grade graduation!" For my mother, these physical items bring her a sense of security and emotional connection. For me, I may not hold on to physical stuff too tightly, but I relentlessly hold on to people. I have a very hard time ending relationships and letting people go, even though some ebb and flow is a natural part of the world's cycles.

Have you ever noticed a desire to hold on to something—whether it's clothing, a house, a job, money, or a relationship—even when it no longer serves you? We can get stuck holding on to less tangible objects, such as habits, reputations, ideas, or grudges. Yogis call this tendency "grasping." Our grasping creates a sticky quality, when we become attached to things working out just the way that we want so that we can look and feel good.

When we grasp, we attach our sense of identity or security to something

"For those who have no inclination to steal, the truly precious is at hand."
—Sutra 2.37

"Freedom from wanting unlocks the real purpose of existence."
—Sutra 2.39

outside of us. We mistakenly believe that holding on to the external object, idea, or person will bring us safety and worthiness.

This is an example of avidya, or the "great mistake." When we make the great mistake, we forget that worthiness and groundedness can only be found inside us. When we pause, breathe, and go inside, we find a true connection to our wholeness that is resilient and unchanging. From this space, we can let go of trying to control the world around us.

In *The Yoga Sutras*, Patanjali outlines external observances for relating to the world. These include non-stealing *(asteya)* and non-grasping *(aparigraha)*.

PRACTICE

- ▶ Come into a comfortable, tall seat.
- ▶ Soften your face, throat, and eyes.
- ▶ Take a few slow breaths.
- ▶ What if nothing needed to be different, right now?
- ▶ What would it feel like to be free from wanting?

REFLECTION

▶ Have you ever wanted to take something? (In addition to a physical object or money, this could include someone's time or ideas.)

▶ Why have you felt "sticky" about something (a person, object, idea, etc.)?

▶ What do you feel you are protecting by controlling that thing?

▶ What were you trying to gain from holding on to it?

▶ Consider a time in the past that you felt attached to something or someone. What was the result?

▶ Consider a time that you let something go. What was the result?

20. SADNESS AND DISCONNECTION

Anava Mala

According to tantric philosophy, you are a wondrous expression of the unfolding of divine universal consciousness. At its core, there is no separation between self and other, and we are all one.

So, if we're so great, why do we feel so bad?

At the core of human existence, is a fundamental sense of restlessness, emptiness, or longing. Tantric yogis call this feeling of incompleteness *anava mala*, and it is related to our hearts. Anava mala is one of the three core misperceptions that keep us from recognizing our own worthiness. Rather than remember our connection to our source, we often feel anxious, lacking, sad, and disconnected.

Because of anava mala, we try to fill this "inner hole" with resources from the external world. To feel better, we may engage is tactics like buying stuff, taking a prestigious job, eating ice cream, or clinging to unfulfilling romantic relationships. A good friend of mine often jokes that she likes to "eat her feelings." In addition to eating my own feelings (or occasionally drinking them) when I feel sad or lost, I overwork. Accomplishing something gives me the sense that I deserve to be loved. But soon enough, the glow of achievement wears off, and I'm scampering for the popcorn, wine, or to-do list to feel okay.

No matter how much we shore up our experience with stuff outside of us, this feeling of lack is simply part of being human, and it can only be truly filled through patient inner work.

In a way, this is excellent news because we no longer have to worry that something is wrong with us when we feel lost or sad. The even better news: these feelings of unworthiness are a misperception, not reality. When we feel this inner restlessness, we can smack our own foreheads and think, "Ah-ha! There's anava mala, at it again." We can then take a deep breath and devote time to reconnecting to our own inner resources.

PRACTICE

▶ Come into a comfortable, tall seat.

▶ Soften your face, throat, and eyes.

▶ Close your eyes.

▶ Take a few slow, deep breaths.

▶ Notice the rising and falling of your thoughts and feelings.

▶ Allow all the thoughts and feelings to have space to come and go. (Crying in meditation is just fine.)

▶ Notice that, given space and presence, even intense feelings will shift and change into something else.

▶ Connect to the space that is watching these sensations arise: your presence (or self, or witness).

▶ From this inner space beyond the thinking, in this moment, is anything really lacking?

REFLECTION

▶ How do you usually try to fill your inner feeling of scarcity? What are your favorite tactics?

▶ As you move through the day, can you catch yourself before you try to fill the void? We're usually so good at avoiding this inner feeling that we cover it up before we even notice it. Try to pause and stay in the uncomfortable feeling for 10 breaths before "fixing" it.

▶ As you experience your sensations, thoughts, and feelings, can you also connect to the presence that holds space for all of these experiences?

21. COMPARISON AND JEALOUSY

Mayiya Mala

There's a saying: "A rich man is the one who earns five dollars more than his neighbor."

We continually compare ourselves to others, jockeying to see if we measure up. We compare everything: our appearance, success, good fortune, likeability—the list goes on and one. Our culture, rooted in competition and capitalism, encourages these judgmental feelings. Standards for beauty and achievement are impossible to meet. When we compete with Photoshop beauty and celebrity wealth, it's hard to look good by comparison. And our constant feeling of lack makes the economic world go round; after all, the best marketing creates a need you didn't know you had, then sells you the solution to fix it!

Given that someone out there will always be prettier, richer, thinner, and more successful, how are we supposed to feel good about ourselves?

According to tantric yoga, this feeling of separateness and comparison is called *mayiya mala*. Related to the mind, it is one of three core misperceptions that keep us from recognizing our connection to everything around us. In the tantric worldview, we are all part of one divine whole. Given that we spend so much time labeling and differentiating things, this may seem a little counterintuitive. But it all depends on your point of view. If you imagine the world from the point of view of quantum physics, we are all immersed in a seething, connected form of particles. In the same way, the tantra affirm that — despite the seeming differences — we're part of one continuity from the highest perspective.

To account for the seeming differences, tantra recognizes forces at play that keep us from recognizing our intrinsic connection. Mayiya mala creates the experience of subject and object, where I perceive myself as being separate from you. Once that happens, then the comparisons start. This confusion leads to feelings of jealousy, anger, and unworthiness.

The good news: it's normal to feel this way. Mayiya mala is an intrinsic part of the universal order. The even better news: if we practice reconnecting to our true nature, then the apparent separations between us and everything else will start to dissolve.

....

"A human being is a part of the whole, called by us universe, a part limited in time and space. He experiences himself, his thoughts, and feelings as something separated from the rest — a kind of optical delusion of his consciousness. This delusion is a kind of prison for us, restricting us to our personal desires and to affection for a few persons nearest to us. Our task must be to free ourselves from this prison by widening our circle of compassion to embrace all living creatures and the whole of nature in its beauty."

—Albert Einstein

....

PRACTICE FOR RECOGNITION OF INTERCONNECTION

▶ Take a comfortable seat.

▶ Take a few deep breaths and close your eyes.

▶ Focus on your breath.

▶ As you do, begin to notice that the air you are breathing connects you intimately with the outer world.

▶ With every inhale, you bring the world into you (oxygen from trees, plants, etc.).

▶ With every exhale, you give back to the world.

▶ Can you extend your vision, imagining the collective breathing of all the humans, plants, and animals around you?

▶ Feel your participation with the great breath of the earth.

PRACTICE FOR RECOGNITION OF PERSPECTIVE

▶ Take a comfortable seat.

▶ Take a few deep breaths and close your eyes.

▶ Consider another person who has caused you to experience jealousy.

- ▶ For a moment, indulge in all the feelings of comparison that come up for you.

- ▶ After a minute, let that go and take a few deep breaths.

- ▶ Consider this person again.

- ▶ This time, focus on all your similarities (experiences, passions, vulnerabilities, physical similarities—anything).

- ▶ Stay with this contemplation for a few minutes.

- ▶ How did that feel?

REFLECTION

- ▶ When and why do I find myself comparing myself with others?

- ▶ What do I get out of being "better"?

- ▶ What do I get out of being "worse"?

- ▶ What practices help me find connection rather than disconnection?

22. WHY IS MY MIND SO CRAZY?

Parts of the Mind

Does your mind sometimes spin out of control?

The good news is that you're in very good company. The even better news is that yogis have been studying the mind for thousands of years. By understanding how the mind works, we are better equipped to use the mind as a tool, rather than let it run the show.

We all have voices in our heads that are all vying for control. By identifying "who" is talking, we can determine who to put in the driver's seat.

Here are the major players:

▶ Sense organs: allow you to sense the world around you through touch, hearing, sight, smell, and taste.

▶ *Manas*, the "lower mind," pulls together sensory information and compiles it to create an experience of the world.

▶ *Ahamkara*, the ego, or "I-maker," helps us to distinguish ourselves from the world around us. (I am happy, I am sad, I am a good person, I am an architect, I am a yogi, I am a mother, etc.).

"The mind is a wonderful servant but a terrible master."

—Robin Sharma

Ahamkara attaches our sense of self to an experience.

▶ *Smrti*, one of the *vrittis* (fluctuations of the mind and memor) is the storehouse of our past impressions and experiences and can provide information for how to navigate the present moment. Left on autopilot, smriti will create reactions based on past experiences.

▶ *Buddhi*, higher mind, is the voice of discrimination *(viveka)* and is connected to your higher self.

To illuminate the different parts of our minds, consider this story:

You're finishing up a long day of work and are tired. Your body feels sore, lethargic, and stiff (sense organs). I'm tired, you think (ego). You open the freezer and see (sense organ) a frozen pizza. It's your roommate's and she's out of town. She's told you to have whatever you like (memory).

Inside your mind, your ego and your memory have a quick confab. Do I like pizza? your ego asks your memory. Yes!, memory replies.

Yay! says ego, and tells your hand to grab the pizza.

Wait!, shouts a new voice. Ego and memory turn around to see buddhi running forward. They regard buddhi suspiciously because buddhi isn't always the most fun person at the party.

Memory buddhi asks, What happens after you eat pizza? Memory pauses and shuffles its feet a bit, but is willing to answer honestly and thoroughly when asked the right question: I don't tolerate gluten or cheese very well, and I feel bloated and my tummy hurts.

So should we really eat this pizza? Buddhi asks. After all, there's also a nice salad in the fridge.

Ego stamps its feet. But I worked hard and I deserve it! I need to have some pleasure in my life! Waaaaaaaaaahhhhh! And ego throws a temper tantrum.

Buddhi finally says sharply, Ego, get a grip! You know you feel like crap after eating pizza, and you've been whining lately about how your yoga pants feel tight. So stop whining already and leave the pizza alone!

And under the influence of buddhi, they step away from the pizza, and decide to have the nice salad after all. And after eating, ego smugly says, I'm so glad that I made that smart decision. I was right all along.

REFLECTION

▶ Which part of your mind is usually in the driver's seat?

▶ How can you tell which part of your mind is talking to you?

▶ What practices can you undertake so that buddhi has room to share its point of view?

23. FOR SURRENDER

Isvara Pranidhana

Sometimes, you have to let go.

In *The Yoga Sutras*, Patanjali outlines three components to kriya yoga, the yoga of action.

Tapas can be literally translated as "heat." Swami Satchidananda translates it as "accepting pain as help for purification," but I prefer the definition, "the willingness to endure intensity for the sake of transformation. Tapas incites us to engage our willpower, fire up our effort, and to embrace discomfort to move forward.

Svadhyaya is self-study, the willingness to frankly and deeply look at ourselves.

And the third component, *isvara pranidhana* — the yoga of action — is a willingness to surrender to the highest.

....

Tapah svadhyayesvara pranidhanani kriya yogah

"Accepting pain as help for purification, study of spiritual books, and surrender to the Supreme Being constitute Yoga in practice."

—Sutra 2.1

....

For many of us, surrender is the most challenging aspect of kriya yoga. In a world that demands achievement, independence, and forward movement, it can seem easier to embrace discomfort than to practice letting go. We are taught that we are the architects of our destiny, but this fails to accommodate for circumstances that arise beyond our control.

Learning to let go is not the same thing as giving up. Recognizing the limits of our personal responsibility is not the same thing as relinquishing accountability. There comes a point when we have done what we can, and our only next step is to "let go and let God." When we surrender to the highest, we are mindfully giving our trust over to something greater than ourselves.

PRACTICE

▶ Take time each day to focus lightly on your breath.

▶ Sit quietly and then let yourself feel your breath moving in and out of your body.

▶ Give yourself over to your body's natural rhythm and trust your innate intelligence.

REFLECTION

▶ What is my relationship to surrender?

▶ What is my relationship to control?

▶ What do I lose by letting go?

▶ What do I gain?

▶ How did letting go in the past turn out?

24. PURIFICATION

Sauca

Cleaning out closets, engaging in a juice fast, avoiding sugar, unplugging from technology are all examples of *sauca*, or "purification." Purification practices help us to create clarity and simplicity. When our lives feel overloaded — with material stuff or too much to do — our minds can start running on the hamster wheel. Engaging in a purification practice helps us cleanse the distractions from our lives so that we can create a clear and more open space.

Practically speaking, it's hard to practice yoga or calm our minds when our bodies don't feel well. If we're recovering from a hangover, stressed out, or have eaten heavy food, it's harder to clear our minds and feel connected to our inner wholeness.

Through the practiced of sauca, we can become more conscious and caring stewards of our bodies, so that they can support us to live vibrant, sustainable lives.

PRACTICE

Engaging in purification practices can also take into account our mental and emotional health. In addition to physical practices, sauca practices could include the following:

- ▶ Clear your calendar.
- ▶ Fast from social media.
- ▶ Donate stuff you no longer use.
- ▶ Drink enough water.
- ▶ Have a good, cleansing sweat.
- ▶ Eat nourishing foods.
- ▶ Fast intermittently.
- ▶ Take space for yourself.
- ▶ Exercise.
- ▶ Get good rest.
- ▶ Speak honestly.
- ▶ Unplug from technology.
- ▶ Create good boundaries in relationships.
- ▶ Clear toxic energy from your life.
- ▶ Develop new, healthy habits.

REFLECTION

▶ Where in your life do you feel cluttered or overwhelmed?

▶ Where in your life would you like to create more simplicity or clarity?

▶ What is one small step you can take to make that change?

▶ Can you make any dietary changes that will serve your overall health?

25. CONTENTMENT

Santosha

What is your relationship to contentment?

Santosha is one of the *niyamas*, which are guidelines for relating more graciously with ourselves. Santosha invites us to practice "being with what is," rather than fighting constantly against the world. When we practice contentment, we begin to soften to the present moment. Finding the space to be, rather than do, allows us to receive and immerse ourselves in the world as it is. We drop our agendas, and stop trying to exact control on the circumstances — and people — around us. By giving ourselves space, we also give others room to be as they are.

When we are not content, we are often fighting to change the world. Although a wholesome zeal is healthy, focusing only on our goals means we can only see our own agenda. We're like a horse with blinders on; although helpful for getting to our destination, we may miss the sights and side routes along the way.

When we drop our control strategies, we can take in the vista of our whole experience and see outside the tunnel vision of our own wants and desires. We discover the small wonders of this present moment. Being present brings us many gifts — the air on our

> "Contentment brings unsurpassed joy."
> —Sutra 2.42

skin, the feel of our breath, the sound of the wind—that we may miss when we are focused on doing.

Contentment is the antidote of regret, or self-blame, which keeps us locked in the past. Regret is a way of trying to control our history; we believe that if we feel badly enough, we can somehow change something that already happened. When we blame ourselves for something—a relationship, a dream deferred, a misstep—we are looking back with 20/20 hindsight, rather than acknowledging that we did the best we could at the time. Blame keeps us locked in the drama of the experience. Although practicing contentment doesn't alleviate our accountability, it gives us the space to learn from what we did and move forward.

PRACTICE

You can practice this walking meditation seated if you prefer:

▶ Without a particular agenda or destination, go for a walk.

▶ As you do, immerse yourself in the sights and senses of the world around you.

▶ Can you experience the world just as it is, curious about what it will bring you?

REFLECTION

▶ In what areas of your life do you struggle with contentment? What are you protecting by not allowing things to be?

▶ A wonderful way to cultivate contentment is to start a daily gratitude practice by listing at least five things for which you are grateful.

▶ Write down any unresolved areas of self-blame from the past. What did you learn from experience that you treasure?

26. HAPPINESS AND SUFFERING

Avidya

Avidya, "non-seeing," is the fundamental obstacle to happiness and self-awareness. In sutra 2.5, Patanjali explains that avidya is seeing the impermanent as permanent, the impure as pure, and the non-self as the self.

Have you ever completely identified yourself with something, like a job, skill, or place you lived—and then lost it?

One of my friends was a professional Irish step dancer. She devoted her entire childhood and adolescence to her dance career. By the time she was 20, she had fractured both her shins and was no longer able to dance. She was devastated. Dancing was her life. Who was she, if not a dancer?

In this instance, she suffered from a case of mistaken identity. She had believed that something impermanent—her identity as a dancer, and the resilience of her body—was permanent. We all do this in some way. Perhaps you attach your sense of self-esteem to a job and your achievements, or to your appearance, health, or relationships. When these elements change—as they will and must—we feel as if the ground has fallen out from underneath us. Although it's normal, and part of the joy of being alive to experience and enjoy these things while we can, Patanjali cautions that we suffer when we become overly attached to things that will inevitably change. When we remember that they are impermanent, we can hold them more lightly. We can savor their ephemeral beauty rather than take them for granted.

PRACTICE

▶ Take a tall, comfortable seat.

▶ Enjoy a few deep, easy breaths.

▶ Watch your thoughts as they arise and dissipate.

▶ Rather than get caught up in the content, be an observer.

▶ Giving time and space for each question, consider:

  ▶ Who is the watcher? Who is looking out of your eyes?

  ▶ Five years ago, who was looking out of your eyes?

  ▶ Ten years ago, who was looking out of your eyes?

  ▶ When you were 10, who was looking out of your eyes?

  ▶ When you were a baby, who was looking out of your eyes?

This is the self.

REFLECTION

▶ When in the past have you suffered because you mistook the impermanent for permanent?

▶ Make a list of what is most important to you right now. Are these things permanent or impermanent?

▶ How might recognizing their impermanence make them more precious?

▶ Spend time in nature and notice the natural cycles around you that contain beginnings, middles, endings, and new beginnings.

27. SELF-STUDY

Svadhyaya

One of the components of kriya yoga (yoga of action) is *svadhyaya*, or self-study. Patanjali also lists svadhyaya as one of the niyamas, or internal observances.

Svadhyaya operates on two levels: becoming aware of our own conditioning, and recognizing our own true nature.

Becoming aware of our conditioning increases our accountability for how we navigate the world.

Before I was married, I didn't know how to engage in conflict. My ex-husband was much more accustomed to expressing what he wanted—vigorously and passionately. When my marriage encountered problems and he started getting loud, I shut down and went silent. Only through studying our dynamic over time did I realize I had a blind spot when it came to expressing myself in conflict.

We are only consciously aware of a small part of our conditioning. If you'd asked me before my marriage how I would be in an emotional and psychological conflict, I would have thought of myself as a strong,

Sva: self

Dhyaya: contemplate

grounded human who could hold her own. Personal circumstances, however, exposed a different and deeper pattern. Although this exposure was painful, this awareness enabled me to learn more about myself, and do the work to consciously learn a new communication pattern.

Think of yourself as an iceberg. Although you may have a conscious sense of the tip of your own iceberg, you are unconscious of the vast majority of the iceberg that glides beneath the surface. And clearly, what's beneath the water will determine how you operate and where you go. By watching how you interact with the world, you can begin to see your conditioning more clearly. Through the practice of svadhyaya, you can make conscious choices about how you want to relate to yourself and others.

Your conditioning is not your destiny; through the power of consciousness, you have the ability to make new choices that uphold who you want to be.

The second layer of svadhyaya is recognition of your own true nature. Becoming mindful of your conditioning can help you improve your behavior, but it will not necessarily support your spiritual liberation. If you think of your personality as a house that you live in, then evolving your conditioning is a little like renovating and redecorating your house. Liberation is like leaving the house entirely.

Spiritual liberation requires detangling your habitual identification of self with your ego/personality, and learning to recognize self as the consciousness and awareness that lies within you. Imagine you are a drop of water in the ocean; spiritual liberation involves recognizing your connection with the entire ocean. Practices such as meditation and studying spiritual books can help us to connect more deeply with the self as awareness.

REFLECTION

▶ What does your yoga practice reveal about you? (Do you tend to dial it back, or "push through"? Do you prefer movement or stillness? Music or silence?)

▶ What is the relationship between vulnerability and growth?

▶ When you encounter discomfort, what do you do?

▶ Reflect upon your day: What did your choices reveal about who you are?

▶ What are your go-to books for feeling connected and elevated?

28. DISLIKE

Dvesha

Where does dislike come from?

When I was in college, my roommate took me out for sushi. I'd never had sushi before and I hated the new tastes and textures. I couldn't understand what she liked about it and was very reluctant to try it again.

According to the yogis, the origin of aversion, or *dvesha*, is simple. We dislike something we associate with an unpleasurable experience.

Animals are often trained through stimulus response: if they get a treat, they repeat a behavior; if the response is negative, they will shun the behavior. Humans aren't any different: we generally want to avoid experiences that have been unpleasant. Over time, we accumulate a storehouse of memories that train our likes and dislikes. After all, you only have to touch a hot stove once.

> "Aversion is that which follows identification with painful experiences."
> —Sutra 2.8

Although learning to avoid danger is a survival skill, not all aversion is helpful. After all, going to the gym or having a hard conversation isn't pleasant, but it is good for us. Part of our yoga practice is to become aware of our learned conditioning so we may make conscious choices. When we recognize that our present perception is being filtered through a lifetime of previous experiences, we can be more alert to when the past falsely colors our point of view.

A few weeks after I had my first sushi experience, I tried it again. Turns out that I love sushi. If I hadn't been willing to test my assumptions about my initial aversion, I would have missed out on one of my favorite foods.

REFLECTION

▶ When a sense of aversion or dislike arises, become curious.

▶ Can you remember the first time you experienced this dislike?

▶ If the present moment were a clear slate, might you experience it differently?

▶ Do you have any aversions you wish to reframe or change?

29. FEAR OF CHANGE

Abhinivesa

Human nature abhors uncertainty. Even when change is for the better, we balk at changing our life. Our instinctive impulse to hunker down and endure is why many of us stay in relationships, jobs, and situations that don't really serve us or allow us to fully thrive.

I was in a relationship that made me very unhappy. When I spoke about my situation with my friends, breaking up was the obvious solution. But as soon as I started to take action, I became consumed by crippling panic. My logical mind crumpled in the anxiety that arose in the face of ending my relationship.

Abhinivesa is the fear of death. It reflects a primal desire to cling to what is habitual and to avoid change or loss. One of the obstacles *(kleshas)* to self-realization, abhinivesa is said to be powerful, even in the wise.

Find comfort in the fact that it is normal to be afraid of change. It's normal to want to hold on. It doesn't have to feel good to be right. Ending my relationship felt terrible, but ultimately it was the best thing to do.

> "Clinging to life is instinctive and self-perpetuating, even for the wise."
>
> —Sutra 2.9

When we are confronted with change, it's natural to want to freeze or change course. Rather than react, we can practice holding space for our discomfort. When we do, we may begin to recognize something within us that is whole and safe. When we connect with this steady sense of awareness, we anchor our awareness in a deeper connection that will help us to sustain the choices that align with our highest selves.

PRACTICE

- ▶ Come into a comfortable seat.

- ▶ Take a few deep, expansive breaths.

- ▶ As you settle, notice your thoughts and feelings.

- ▶ Allow them to come and go.

- ▶ Connect to the space of the witness, or observer, of your experience.

- ▶ From this perspective, are you safe in this moment?

- ▶ From this perspective, are you whole in this moment?

REFLECTION

▶ What is your emotional relationship to change?

▶ Consider a time when your world "fell apart." How did you navigate the chaos?

▶ Does anything in your life need to end? What has stood in the way?

▶ What practices support you to stay connected to a sense of safety and wholeness?

30. CULTIVATING STABILITY

Muladhara Chakra

Part of the subtle body system, chakras are places in the body where energy is particularly condensed. Although there are energy centers all through the body, the seven primary chakras run along the spine, from pelvis to crown. Each chakra is associated with a particular element: earth, water, fire, air, ether, light, thought. Earth is associated with the first chakra, and thought is associated with the seventh. (However, "higher" chakras aren't better; each is necessary for holistic health.) A modern view of the chakras assigns each governance over different aspects of our experience and assigns each chakra with a different psychological fundamental right.

Situated in the base of the pelvis, *muladhara* ("root") chakra governs our connection with physical reality, materialism, and our bodies. Not surprisingly, it is associated with the element earth and our right to physically exist. As the closest chakra to the ground, it physically relates to our pelvis, legs, and organs of elimination. Someone who has a strong connection to this element may be said to have their "feet on the ground," or "be grounded," or seem "anchored." They have a strong sense of their physical presence and aren't afraid to take up space.

But too much earth energy can lead to heaviness, lethargy, stubbornness, and inertia. Symptoms of excessive muladhara include physical heaviness, rigidity, hoarding, and materialism. Too little earth energy can be equally problematic; someone may be delusional, ungrounded, or have their "head in the clouds."

PRACTICE

▶ Hold standing yoga poses to cultivate stability in legs and pelvis.

▶ Practice yin yoga to focus on long holds for pelvis and legs.

▶ Do: squats and lunges to energize the legs and pelvis.

▶ Get out in nature.

▶ Stamp feet.

▶ Do visualizations.

▶ On inhale, imagine pulling energy from the center of the earth to the core of your pelvis.

▶ On exhale, send energy from your pelvis down into the earth.

REFLECTION

▶ What is my relationship to my physical body?

▶ How do I feel about "taking up space"?

▶ What is my relationship to material possessions?

▶ Do I have too much earth, too little, or do I feel balanced? If I'm out of balance, what could I do for self-care?

31. CULTIVATING FLOW

Svadhisthana Chakra

Svadhisthana ("sweetness") chakra is the energy center that governs our relationship with flow, sensuality, and our emotions, and is associated with our right to feel. Situated just below the navel, this chakra relates to our urinary and sexual organs (bladder, urethra, ovaries, uterus, prostrate, testicles, penis, vagina). A balanced relationship to this chakra is reflected in a healthy relationship to one's sensuality, sexuality, and feelings.

Svadhisthana is associated with the element water. Water invites a sense of flow, movement, receiving, and letting go. Water needs movement to be healthy; lack of healthy circulation leads to stagnation and disease. Our emotions and sensations are like water; they need space to be felt and to change.

Someone who may have an excess of this energy may have loose boundaries, have difficulty holding space, or feel overrun by their feelings. Someone who experiences a deficiency in this energy may suppress their feelings, be locked up or rigid, or be unavailable to the flow of sensual energy.

PRACTICE

▶ Do flow styles of yoga that focus on movement and breath.

▶ Do yin yoga/hip openers.

▶ Inspire the senses: enjoy eating a delicious food slowly, savoring a beautiful view, or enjoying the sensation of touching different textures.

▶ Slow down and take time to feel.

▶ Spend time emotional journaling and healing.

REFLECTION

▶ What is my relationship to my feelings?

▶ What is my relationship to my sensual nature?

▶ Would I be served by creating stronger boundaries, or do I want to invite more flow?

▶ Do I have too much water, too little, or do I feel balance? If I'm out of balance, what could I do for self-care?

32. CULTIVATING FIRE

Manipura Chakra

Located at the solar plexus, *manipura chakra* is an energy center controlled by the element of fire and is related to willpower and transformation. Manipura controls how we assert the ego in relationship to the world and is related to the right to take action.

Physically, manipura is related to digestion, where fire (acid, bile) is used to transform external material into sustenance. Similarly, manipura relates to our ability to emotionally "digest" and process our experiences.

When people have excessive fire energy, they may be controlling, overbearing, and arrogant. If they have too little fire energy, they may lack a sense of self and be overly accommodating.

PRACTICE

- ▶ Do hot yoga or power yoga.

- ▶ Focus on the abdomen with twists and core yoga poses.

- ▶ Focus on cardio or weights, heat building, core exercises, boxing or martial arts.

- ▶ Get a good sweat in a sauna.

- ▶ Focus intensely on one thing.

- ▶ Communicate needs and desires clearly.

REFLECTION

- ▶ What is my relationship to my own fire and sense of self?

- ▶ What is my relationship to my willpower?

- ▶ Am I able to assert my own needs, wants, and desires?

- ▶ Am I able to listen to others?

- ▶ Do I have too much fire, too little, or do I feel balanced? If I'm out of balance, what could I do for self-care?

33. GIVING AND RECEIVING LOVE

Anahata Chakra

Anahata chakra is our heart center and is located in the very middle of the chakra system. It is the midway point between the lower three chakras (relating to the energy of the material world) and the etheric elements (relating to energy of the spiritual world). Anahata is the bridge between the earth and sky and is associated with the right to love.

Anahata means "unstruck," which is a reminder that our innermost heart is pure, untouched, and free. Governed by air and movement, anahata is related physically to our lungs, heart, and arms. Anahata's energy is made physical through how we reach out and touch the world.

Anahata is about negotiating balance; our heart chakra governs how we both receive and express love, just as our lungs receive and exhale air. If we have too much air energy, we may lose ourselves in someone else, lack boundaries, and "give ourselves away." If we are lacking in this center, we may withhold love or be stingy in our loving expression. When healthy and in balance, anahata governs our ability to engage in healthy and nourishing exchange: to give as well as receive from others.

PRACTICE

▶ Do heart openers or side body-opening yoga poses.

▶ Pranayama opens the ribs and expands the breath.

▶ Focus on heart-centered meditations.

▶ Donate your time or energy to a good cause.

▶ Do acts of kindness for others.

▶ Create a list of everything and everyone you are grateful for.

▶ Observe the mystery of the world with awe on nature walks or in the night sky.

REFLECTION

▶ What is my relationship to my own heart?

▶ What is my relationship to self-love?

▶ Are there areas (or relationships) in my life where I feel out of balance in giving and receiving?

▶ Do I struggle to give, or do I struggle to receive?

▶ How can I make space to focus on my own needs?

▶ What practices can I use to self-care for my heart?

34. COMMUNICATION

Vishuddha Chakra

The throat chakra, *vishuddha* governs our self-expression and our right to speak. Located in the sternal notch, the element of vishuddha is ether and is physically related to our vocal cords, mouth, sinuses, and throat. Ether is the most refined of the five elements; with vishuddha, we have left the more visceral energies of the lower chakras and moved closer to the refined energy of consciousness.

Vishuddha governs our conscious self-expression. Although this energy may manifest in how we literally speak, it may also emerge in how we share our voice through our work, art, and hobbies.

When the energy in this chakra is excessive, we may talk incessantly and over-share a point of view. We might inundate our audience with words, and find it challenging to listen to others. When the energy of this center is undernourished, we may find it challenging to share ourselves authentically, find expression, or speak our truth. When vishuddha is well balanced, we are able to powerfully articulate who we are in the world, while at the same time leaving space for others to be heard.

PRACTICE

▶ Do chanting, mantra, kirtan.

▶ Try twists (turning head), fish, or shoulder stand.

▶ Sing or speak in public.

▶ Spend time writing creatively.

▶ Share your feelings in a safe space.

▶ Do expressive arts: painting, art, dance, free movement, acting, etc.

REFLECTION

▶ What is my relationship to my own communication?

▶ What is the quality of my speech?

▶ What is the quality of my listening?

▶ How can I nourish my own authentic expression?

35. VISION

Ajna Chakra

Located at our "third eye" between the eyebrows, *ajna chakra* is the energy center for visualization. Related to our optic nerve and our brain, the element of ajna is light and its right is to see. At the third eye, we have moved past the five gross elements (earth, water, fire, air, ether) of the first five chakras and now are firmly in the realm of etheric energy.

Ajna governs our vision and imagination. Humans have a rare and extraordinary ability to conceive of ideas, images, and metaphors beyond the realm of the five senses or the present moment. Our imagination enables us to problem solve and innovate beyond the bounds of our current knowledge, leading to technology, art, spirituality, science, and culture.

When this energy center is well balanced, we have a creative springboard to imagine new possibilities, create a vision for our future, and develop plans and goals that extend into the future. However, when this energy is excessive, we may get caught up in delusion, fantasy, anxiety, or paranoia. An uncontrolled mind may run wild with worry or distraction. When ajna chakra is deficient, then we may feel trapped in old ideas, habits, or conditioning.

PRACTICE

▶ Meditate and visualize.

▶ Do child's pose with forehead on a block.

▶ Do activities that stimulate the mind, like games, puzzles, riddles, math, or coloring books.

▶ Read elevating books.

▶ Entertain and debate new ideas.

▶ Create goals for the future, and visualize your ideal life.

▶ Enjoy cultural appreciation by listening to music, or visiting museums, ballet, theater, the symphony, etc.

REFLECTION

▶ What is my relationship to my own imagination?

▶ What is my relationship to my thoughts and the stories in my head?

▶ Am I able to manifest my ideas into reality?

▶ Am I open to dreaming new possibilities?

36. SPIRITUALITY

Sahasrara

The crown chakra, *sahasrara*, is the energetic center that governs our relationship with a higher spiritual power. Physically, this chakra is related to the brain, as well as the space above the head, and its right is to know. The most etheric of the chakras, this center's associated element is thought, and it enables us to step beyond the bounds of our individual identity to connect with universal consciousness. Through sahasrara, we participate in our relationship with the divine.

If we are excessive in this spiritual energy, we may not seem grounded in earthly reality. Someone who is connected to sahasrara without the stability of the more visceral chakras may be an otherworldly mystic or ascetic who leaves behind earthly energies to commune with their God. Someone who is deficient in this energy may not experience their connection to something bigger than themselves. They may find it hard to experience awe and wonder, or may feel shut off from spiritual connection.

Someone who is well balanced in this energy will be able to experience a rich and growing connection to the divine, while keeping their feet firmly rooted on the earth.

PRACTICE

▶ Meditate or visualize.

▶ Work on your headstand or headstand prep.

▶ Engage in elevating spiritual conversations.

▶ Read spiritual books.

▶ Listen to mantra.

▶ Engage in experiences that create awe and wonder, like nature walks or stargazing..

▶ Spend quiet time in introspection and self-inquiry.

REFLECTION

▶ What is my relationship to my spirituality?

▶ Where do I experience awe and wonder?

▶ How can I create more space for the divine in my daily life?

37. TRANSFORMATION AND ALCHEMY

Hatha Yoga

We might associate the word *hatha* with a softer style of yoga practice, but the word means "forceful." Historically, hatha is a school of yoga that developed in the Middle Ages. The goal for hatha yogis was to create an "adamantine" body that was strong enough to withstand the forces of transformation. To this end, they developed a rich array of body-based practices such as *asana* (postures), *pranayama* (breathing practice), *kriyas* (cleansing techniques), *mudra* (seals), *bandhas* (energetic locks), and *drishti* (gazing points) to cleanse, intensify, and focus the power of the body.

Hatha yoga emerged from the philosophical roots of tantric yoga, and was also influenced by the practice of alchemy. A forerunner to chemistry, practitioners of alchemy sought to transmute base metals and substances into precious and refined substances like gold. Although alchemists pursued this work literally, hatha yogis worked metaphorically to eradicate impurities in their bodies and minds. Thus purified, they were more easily able to enter states of meditation and connect with the absolute.

In this same way, our modern yoga practice is a process of conscious transformation. Every time we arrive at the mat, or our meditation seat, we deliberately create a sacred space in which to shift our experience. Some of these changes are physical (open hamstrings, stronger core), but the most profound shifts are mental, emotional, and spiritual.

As hatha yogis, we are the living continuation of this lineage. We are modern day alchemists, evolving and refining our lives with every practice.

REFLECTION

► What in your life right now requires transformation? (Consider attitude, material possessions, relationships, habits.)

► What will you gain?

► How can your practice (asana, pranayama, meditation, or mindfulness) support your transformation?

38. ANGER

Kali

Hindu philosophy is replete with epic tales of gods, goddesses, and magical creatures. Rather than be viewed literally as gods, they are metaphorical figures that provide relatable access points to the various aspects of the divine. Each figure has its own temperament and energetic qualities; by connecting to this aspect of the divine, the devotee is able to call up the essence of its energy.

The goddess Kali is the fierce, dark mother. She is terrifying in her aspect, having red eyes and wearing a necklace of severed heads. She is the most powerful aspect of the goddess, and is evoked when it is time for necessary destruction. Her anger is just, uncontrolled, and undefeatable. She is like a raging fire, purifying and destroying what is in its path to make way for a rebirth. Although Kali is fearsome, she is also worshipped for her fierce love and protection.

Ultimately, anger is protective in nature. It arises from a deep, passionate love to protect something beloved to us. Many of us have been taught to suppress our anger as "non-yogic" or not "nice." Kali reminds us that divine anger can be a powerful vehicle for justice and transformation:

▶ Kali is the energy we call upon to break off a dysfunctional relationship, or say hard things.

▶ Kali is the rage we embrace to uphold our boundaries and protect what is ours.

- Kali is the energy that says, "Stop being nice! Stand up for yourself!"
- Kali is the power that knows when death is the greatest form of kindness.

Although anger can be righteous, it must be managed responsibly so that its blaze is cleansing rather than destructive. Our anger is a sign that something needs to change; it is not a justification for bad behavior. Powerful feelings need to be processed and examined so that we can take action from our highest values. Conscious and accountable anger can provide the energy we need to make positive change. Wildfires are sometimes necessary to burn away the underbrush and make way for new growth.

"Bitterness is like cancer. It eats upon the host. But anger is like fire. It burns it all clean."

—Maya Angelou

REFLECTION

▶ What is your relationship to your own anger (consider that emotions such as irritation and frustration are forms of anger)?

▶ Recall a time that you were angry. What was your anger protecting or upholding?

▶ What kind of self-reflection process would help you listen to your anger and use it in service of good?

▶ Observe as feelings of irritation, frustration, and anger arise. What are these feelings protecting? When you examine your feelings, would giving voice to your anger support your highest values or is your anger pointing to something you personally need to work on and process?

▶ Is there anything in your life you need to end?

39. PLAY

Lila, Iccha-Skakti

In the beginning, there was Brahman (universal consciousness). Brahman was all that there was. Except for one other creature.

Lila approached Brahman and asked, rather mischievously, "Do you want to play a game?"

Brahman perked up. Why yes, he did.

"Okay," said Lila, "Go ahead and create the entire cosmos. Planets, stars, creatures...everything."

Brahman went into action and did as she suggested. He created the entire cosmos: planets, stars, and creatures.

"Alright," said Lila, "Great! Now cut yourself up into little pieces and put a little bit of yourself into everything that you have created."

Brahman looked at her doubtfully.

"Trust me, this is going to be great," Lila assured him.

So, Brahman, cut himself up into all the little pieces, and he put a little bit of himself — universal consciousness — into every single thing.

"Wonderful!" exclaimed Lila, clapping her hands. "Now...go find yourself!"

In tantric philosophy, *lila* means, "divine play," which describes the ultimate game of the universe. According to tantra, the great singularity of the shiva-shakti (universal consciousness and the energy of manifestation) chose to limit its own power so that it could experience manifestation (the physical world) in all its diversity of forms.

Another way to think of this: consider the big bang. Before the big bang, everything in the universe was encapsulated in a pure point of energy-matter-consciousness (according to yogis, this is shiva-shakti). As soon as the big bang occurred, the universe expanded and began to cool. It became limited in its own power, subject to laws of gravity, time, and physics. Only as the universe cooled could the myriad potential forms within that original singularity be expressed. Stars, planets, and life appeared.

From this perspective, the universe is the fabric of universal consciousness *(shiva)*, expressing itself in the manifest universe *(shakti)* through lila to experience the multiplicity in all its forms. One of those forms is you.

This is related to a concept called *iccha-shakti*, which is the divine creative urge for self-expression. Everything in the universe is in a state of expressing itself and its nature. Because we are a part of the universe, we can participate in this dance by consciously choosing to engage in joy and self-expression, simply for the joy of being who we really are.

REFLECTION

▶ What is your relationship to play?

▶ What is the benefit of play?

▶ Where can you cultivate more play and expression in your life?

40. EMBRACING EXPANSION AND CONTRACTION

Spanda

The universe is an expression of divine vibration, called *spanda*.

Everything is in a phase of expansion or contraction. Tides flow, the moon waxes and wanes, flowers bloom and die, we sleep and then we wake.

Both expansion and contraction are essential for life. While expansion facilitates growth, creativity, energy, and expression, contraction creates containment, stability, rest, and quietude. On a practical level, we cannot always be in expansion; we need rest and recovery in order to regain equilibrium.

As creatures of the universe, we are always participating in the flux of spanda. We experience it in a multiplicity of ways:

▶ Our lungs fill with air and then empty.

▶ Our heart fills with blood and then empties.

▶ We gain weight, we lose weight.

▶ We feel happy and expanded, then sad and contracted.

▶ Relationships feel close and intimate, then distant and disconnected.

- We long for connection, then we long to be alone.
- Abundance comes, then abundance goes.
- We give, and we receive.

All these fluctuations are part of the universal heartbeat.

When we are able to recognize that these fluctuations are the essential rhythm of the natural world, we can rest a little easier with the fluctuations that may come.

PRACTICE

- Come into a tall, comfortable seat.
- Take a few centering breaths.
- When your body feels calm and grounded, begin a counted pranayama practice: inhale for an internal count of four; exhale for an internal count of four.
- Repeat 5 to 10 times.
- Explore the feeling of expansion in your yoga practice.
- Focus on the inhalation.
- Stretch the body apart.
- Create space.

- ▶ What do you gain from expanding?
- ▶ Explore the feeling of contraction in your yoga practice.
- ▶ Focus on the exhalation.
- ▶ Pull the body together with muscular strength.
- ▶ Create stability.
- ▶ What do you gain from containment?

REFLECTION

- ▶ Do you have an easier time inhaling (receiving) or exhaling (giving)?
- ▶ How does the energy of expansion support you in life?
- ▶ How does the energy of contraction support you in life?

41. TRUE AND FALSE PERCEPTION

Pramana Vritti | Viparyaya Vritti

The Yoga tradition identifies a few different categories of "mind stuff" or "fluctuations" *(vritti)* to help us recognize and become friends with the workings of our minds.

The yogis were very clear that our perception of reality is limited to the information we can take in through our senses.

Consider these examples:

Although radio waves surround us, we lack the ability to perceive them without a radio.

Dogs can hear higher frequencies and smell far better than we can.

There are numerous wavelengths (infrared, gamma rays, X-rays) that we lack the ability to see.

The first viritti is true perception *(pramana viritti)*. True perception occurs when our idea of the world—that is, what we are experiencing and interpreting through our five senses—accurately matches reality. Although we can never be completely sure that we're correct, we are usually experiencing true perception if one of the following conditions is met:

- ▶ I perceive it directly. (I see a fire and know there is a fire.)
- ▶ Someone I trust has perceived it directly. (My best friend tells me that there is a fire.)
- ▶ There are enough clues that I can make a sensible inference based on my information. (I see smoke, hear fire trucks, and thus know that there is a fire.)

However, our human senses serve us very well, they are limited. And even when we do perceive the world directly, we can mistake our interpretations.

False perception *(viparyaya vritti)* occurs when we perceive the world directly, but interpret it in a way that doesn't align with how things really are.

Consider this traditional yoga story:

> A man is returning to his village at night. By the side of the road, he sees a giant and deadly snake. He runs to his village and warns everyone about the dangerous creature. When the villagers bring a lighted torch to see the snake, they discover that the snake was really just a coiled rope.

In this story, the man has directly perceived something, but his mind has misinterpreted the information. When the light is brought (representing illumination and knowledge), the villagers discover the truth.

We tend to accept our mind's interpretations as the truth. If I see my partner exuberantly embracing someone else, I may leap to conclusions about his fidelity before I find out that his long-lost cousin has come to town. Our minds filter our experiences through our expectations, needs, fears, wants, desires, and values.

We can often see this filtering process clearly in relationships, where we make conclusions about someone's actions based on our prior experiences. If I was hurt in a previous relationship because a partner cheated on me, I may interpret my new partner's actions through a veil of suspicion. If I am eager to make a new relationship work, I may overlook — or not even register — the red flags that keep cropping up.

Patanjali does not judge true perception as good and false perception as bad; he simply points out that our minds are constantly creating stories. By recognizing the nature of our minds, we can stay open to new information and not be so attached to our particular version of reality. We can create space and tolerance to question our assumptions, as well as have more compassion for other people who have different points of view.

As you begin to separate your stories from reality, you will be able to notice the filters (expectations, needs, wants, values, or fears) that are coloring your perception. Through this process, you can engage in a deep process of self-study *(svadhyaya)* and self-recognition. For example, when my partner looks irritated, my habitual reaction is to assume I've done something wrong. However, usually his frown has nothing to do with me and he's deep in thought. By noticing the story I create in my head, I can recognize how quick I am to leap to self-blame. Once I am aware of this conditioned response, I am better able to avoid distorting information in the future.

PRACTICE

▶ Come into a comfortable seat.

▶ Take a few deep, slow breaths.

▶ Slowly tune your attention to your sense of sight. Explore what you are really seeing. Can you see the space with "fresh eyes"? What is here that you've not seen before (or that you have filtered out)?

▶ Continue to explore your sense of sight, or you may cycle through your other senses (hearing, smell, touch, taste), allowing your mind the space and time to register the different kinds of information it can experience.

▶ After several minutes, reflect: on what was in reality that you had been filtering out?

▶ How does this change in perception shift your experience?

REFLECTION

▶ Consider a time that you misinterpreted reality. What did you perceive, and what did you assume? What led the misinterpretation?

▶ As you move through your day, slow down so that you may consider the information your senses are perceiving. See if you can catch yourself creating stories. (For example, my partner looks upset, and I interpret it to mean he is irritated with me.)

▶ Consider what expectations, needs, wants, desires, fears, or values are "coloring" your experience.

42. THE POWER OF IMAGINATION

Vikalpa vritti

The yogis were very clear that our perception of reality is limited to the information that we can take in through our five senses. When we perceive information and it accurately matches reality, it is called true perception. When we perceive information and it does not match reality, it is called false perception. And when we make up something in our minds that is not based in sensory perception, that is imagination *(vikalpa vritti)*.

It's human nature—and one of our gifts—to create stories and imagine new possibilities. Our ability to imagine new possibilities allows us to see a bird and fantasize about the possibility of flight. We taste peanut butter and chocolate and come up with a Reese's Peanut Butter Cup.

However, when left unchallenged, our imagination can take us down a dark path. When we don't recognize that our imagination is not reality, it can lead us to:

▶ Projection

▶ Unfounded expectations

▶ Missing present, real-world opportunities

▶ Unfounded fears

▶ Anxiety

▶ Delusion

▶ Paranoia

My dear friend was in a brief relationship in which she was constantly—and falsely—accused of infidelity. Sometimes her boyfriend would misinterpret events ("You're late! You were clearly out with someone else!") and sometimes he would just completely make up information ("You're thinking about someone else right now!").

Her partner wasn't a bad person, but his imagination was out of control. He wasn't able to see how his fabrications were distorting his perception of reality. Instead, he would be plagued with anxiety based on a deeper inner fear of abandonment and betrayal. Of course, the relationship couldn't withstand the stress of such unfounded fear for very long.

Because it can reveal our subconscious fears and desire, our imagination can provide us with potent and surprising personal insights. A daydream is like a little thought bubble sent up from our subconscious mind; when we're open to observing it, rather than simply believing or dismissing it, it can provide a window into our conditioning.

For example, after my divorce, I was not interested in starting a new relationship or being committed. Yet I would daydream about weddings! Even if I quickly dismissed these fantasies as absurd, the idea was coming from me. By recognizing the fantasy, I could acknowledge that a part of me wanted to marry again. Though our fantasies are certainly not reality, they can provide another avenue for self-study.

Recognizing the potency of imagination, we can also intentionally use it to create a positive experience. Affirmations and positive visualizations are powerful tools that leverage our imagination to support our lives.

PRACTICE

In the morning, pause and create a positive visualization for your day:

▶ Imagine yourself moving through your day with grace and lightness.

▶ Feel yourself how you wish to be as you interact with others.

▶ Imagine yourself moving through some of your daily activities with joy and ease.

▶ If you enjoy affirmations, repeat a positive affirmation to yourself deliberately several times to invite the energy of the affirmation into your life.

At the end of the day, consider how your visualization supported your experience.

REFLECTION:

▶ Are there any common themes to your daydreaming? What fears, needs, wants, desires, or values might they reveal?

▶ When has your imagination been an ally?

▶ When has your imagination been destructive?

▶ Throughout your day, notice when your mind begins to go into fantasy. What triggered vikalpa vritti? What did you get from it?

43. THE POWER OF MEMORY

Smriti Vritti

Memory operates on both a conscious and subconscious level. When we use our memory consciously, we delve into the rich storehouse of our past to gain information that is relevant to the present moment. For example, we might use memory to answer questions such as, When is my friend's birthday? or Where did I leave my keys?

Most of the time, however, our memory operates subconsciously to orient us in the present moment.

Imagine a car ride. The car is your physical body, your soul is the passenger, and the highway is the journey of your life. When you are born, your car is immaculate. The windows of your car are spotless and everything you can see out the windshield is clear and undistorted.

Then you begin your drive. You go everywhere. You drive through the dust of the desert, the pollen of spring flowers. Soon your new car is coated with a thick layer of dust: life has happened.

Now everything you perceive through the windshield is distorted by a thickening layer of grime from the road already traveled. Over time, you may even forget that there is a clear sight line to begin with, because now your world is seen entirely through the distortion of your smudgy, bug-covered windshield.

You see the present through the lens of the past.

As we begin to experience life — whether that experience is good, bad, sad, safe, scary, loving, or unhappy — we relate everything happening now to what has happened before. To keep us safe, our mind creates generalizations, infers meaning, and manufactures patterns.

It's important for human efficiency that this process is largely subconscious. (Just think about everything you would have to remember consciously to drive a car!) However, the subconscious nature of this process means that we will run on autopilot unless we check our assumptions.

On a very practical level, when I see a chair, I know it's a chair because I have learned that some sort of "chair-ness" exists in the world. Chairs have a seat, four legs, and are designed for humans to sit upon. In the world of relationships, I know I've met a good person because he or she acts in ways that I've previously perceived as "good."

Although memory provides us with the wisdom of experience, our previous conditioning makes it challenging for us to have a truly fresh experience. Derailing our assumptions can help us open to new possibilities.

REFLECTION:

▶ Explore what it is like to meet people in your life "freshly" and without expectations. If they were a strangers, how would your interaction change? This exploration can be particularly fun with someone with whom you have a long-standing relationship, like a partner or family member.

▶ Where in your life might memory be holding you back unnecessarily? Is there a way to mindfully check the waters again? As an example, I once took a bad fall out of a handstand, and so I believed for years that I couldn't do it. As it turns out, I was physically strong enough; I had to overcome the story in my mind to move forward.

▶ Consider a strong story from your past that feels negative. Can you rewrite that story now from a more compassionate and supportive point of view?

44. EFFORT AND EASE

Asana

Only one sutra in *The Yoga Sutras* references physical posture. Though it most likely describes the qualities required to sit for meditation or pranayama, it also provides insight for how we can find a "seat" within ourselves.

Patanjali shares that there are two aspects to physical postures: steadiness and ease. A posture that is only steady *(sthira)* or only comfortable *(sukha)* is not asana. Instead, we must seek the balanced action of both strength and ease in our postures.

Most of us have an easier time with one aspect of the practice. Some of us are naturally adept at finding strength, stability, and intensity, although others will gravitate toward ease and letting go. Our yoga practice requires that we bring both of these qualities into balance.

This sutra is an invitation to consider how we balance effort and ease in all aspects of our lives.

....

"Asana is a steady, comfortable posture."

—Sutra 2.46

....

REFLECTION:

▶ What do I gain through ease?

▶ What do I gain through effort?

▶ Which do I tend to favor more instinctively?

▶ How can I cultivate practicing the opposite quality to invite balance into my life?

▶ Yoga practice: through the asana, mindfully invite the qualities for both sthira and sukha into each posture. (The exception: *savasana;* you are invited to completely let go in corpse pose.)

45. THE POWER OF BREATH

Pranayama

Life force *(prana)* is said to ride on the breath. By controlling the breath, we are able to harness this energy and consciously shift our energetic experience. Physiologically, controlling the breath enables us to indirectly access our nervous system. Though we can't consciously regulate our heart rate or blood pressure, we can indirectly access these systems through our breathing.

Interestingly, in Sanskrit, we cannot tell if the word *pranayama* is composed of *prana* and *yama* or *prana* and *ayama*. Pranayama can therefore mean both restraint and expansion of the breath and life force.

In *The Yoga Sutras*, Patanjali enumerates an eight-step process to yoga. Step four is pranayama. The yogis recognized that harnessing the breath is a potent and practical tool for managing the fluctuations of our minds.

PRACTICE

▶ Come into a comfortable seat.

▶ Take a few deep, expansive breaths, then allow your breath to return to its natural cadence.

▶ Sense the quality of your thoughts and your feelings.

▶ Maintaining the ease in your body, inhale for a count of four, then exhale for a count of four.

▶ If your breath is relaxed and without anxiety, you can extend the count (inhale for a count of five, exhale for a count of five, etc.).

▶ If your body can remain relaxed, begin to lengthen the slight pause between the inhale and exhale.

▶ After a few minutes, let the counting go and return to your natural breath.

▶ Again, sense the quality of your thoughts and your feelings.

▶ What has shifted?

REFLECTION

Pranayama can involve a dedicated seated breath practice, but it also includes being aware of your breath as you move through your daily life. As yogis, we can take responsibility for our inner state of energy by using the breath to support our self-regulation:

▶ Throughout your day, pause to notice the different qualities of your breathing (fast, slow, shallow, deep, chest/belly, rough, smooth). Become curious about how different breath qualities may reflect different emotional or mental states.

▶ Begin to incorporate the simple practice of taking three deep, conscious breaths throughout your day to find a personal "reset."

▶ Explore how you can use your breath to support your emotional and mental state:

  ▶ When you are agitated or anxious, practice slowing your breath or lengthening your exhale.

  ▶ When you feel tired, practice lengthening your exhale or taking a few deep sighs to move your energy.

▶ Explore breathing into different parts of your torso: the belly, side ribs, upper chest, upper back, lower back. If you find it hard to access the breath in part of your body, you can enhance your breath awareness by physically stretching that area. For example, if you find it challenging to access breath movement in your upper back, then come into a cat pose and "send" your breath between your shoulder blades.

Keep in mind: there is no one "right" way to breathe. Our body and breathing will naturally shift to accommodate what is needed in the moment. Jogging will require a faster and more rigorous breath pattern than lying in savasana. Our intention is to cultivate flexibility, resiliency, and mindfulness in our breath and our energy.

46. UNDERSTANDING THE SELF: ANXIETY

Vata

Tracing its roots back to the Vedas, Ayurveda an ancient and holistic healing art designed to promote health and longevity, and the sister science to yoga. Healing is achieved through looking at all areas of life: exercise, sleep, activities, massage, self-care practices, and nutrition.

According to Ayurveda and yogic philosophy, the material world consists of five great elements: earth, water, fire, air, ether. Each person's innate disposition *(prakruti)* is determined by how these elements are expressed in their constitution through their *doshas*.

Doshas are composed of two of the five elements. There are three doshas:

▶ Vata: composed of ether and air

▶ Pitta: composed of fire and water

▶ Kapha: composed of water and earth

Although we each are influenced by all three doshas, usually we have one dominant and one subdominant dosha that govern our nature.

Vata

The qualities of vata are similar to those of air and space: light, moving, mobile, quick, cool, dry, spacious, rough, irregular, quick, and changeable. Physically, vata governs digestion, the nervous system, and movement.

People with a balanced vata dosha will be creative, light, agile, charismatic, adventurous, and curious. People who are vata dominant are quick-witted and love excitement.

An excess of vata may be expressed in the following symptoms:

- Nervousness
- Spaciness
- Anxiety, worry
- Delusion
- Feeling hyped up, jittery
- Feeling cold
- Unable to sleep soundly
- Flatulent (too much wind)
- Constipated (too dry)
- Dry skin

REFLECTION:

If you are suffering from too much vata, consider implementing some of the following self-care strategies to counterbalance the energy of this dosha:

- ▶ Engage in warm, slow practices such as hot yin, restorative or hatha yoga.

- ▶ Eat warm, grounding foods (roasted root vegetables, soups.

- ▶ Enjoy a warming sauna.

- ▶ Sit on the earth (grounding).

- ▶ Meditate on connecting to the earth.

- ▶ Avoid stimulants like caffeine.

- ▶ Slow down (breathe slowly, lie down, or take 10 deep, slow breaths).

- ▶ Go to bed early.

- ▶ Lie down with sandbags or blankets on you (grounding).

- ▶ Avoid stimulation, enjoy a retreat from distractions and busyness.

- ▶ Enjoy an oil massage.

- ▶ Avoid stressful situations.

47. UNDERSTANDING THE SELF: ANGER AND CONTROL

Pitta

The qualities of a pitta-dominant personality are similar to those of fire and water (think of a fluidlike oil): fiery, fierce, bright, smart, leading, "type A," energetic, directive. Physically, pitta governs digestion (the energy of fire and transformation).

When pitta is excessive, it may be expressed in the following symptoms:

▶ Domination

▶ Impatience

▶ Punitive behavior

▶ Overly controlling actions

▶ Anger

▶ Acne (too oily, inflamed)

▶ Inflammation/rashes

▶ Ulcers, heartburn (too much acid, heat)

REFLECTION

If you are suffering from too much pitta, consider implementing some of the following self-care strategies to counterbalance the energy of this dosha:

▶ Engage in cooling practices such as flow, yin, restorative or hatha yoga.

▶ Eat cooling foods (cucumbers, melons, fruit).

▶ Rest.

▶ Avoid stress and take a break.

▶ Take cool baths.

▶ Eat regularly.

▶ Enjoy cooling scents or oils (lavender, jasmine, mint).

▶ Focus on pacifying pranayama or meditation practices.

48. UNDERSTANDING THE SELF: LETHARGY AND DEPRESSION

Kapha

The qualities of a kapha-dominant personality are similar to those of earth and water: stable, grounded, rooted, connected, strong, sturdy, thoughtful, compassionate, loyal, and patient.

When kapha is excessive, it may be expressed in the following symptoms:

- Lethargy
- Heaviness
- Slowness
- Weight gain
- Depression
- Stubbornness
- Intractability
- Lack of flow
- Hoarding

REFLECTION:

If you are suffering from too much kapha, consider implementing some of the following self-care strategies to counterbalance the energy of this dosha:

▶ Energize with practices such as power and flow yoga.

▶ Seek out stimulation and excitement.

▶ Get out of the house and into the world.

▶ Eat lightly: enjoy lighter foods and season your food with spice.

▶ Clear your space of clutter and stuff.

▶ Get moving by going for walks or practicing light cardio.

▶ Enjoy warm, stimulating scents like rosemary, eucalyptus or peppermint.

▶ Avoid sweet and heavy foods.

▶ Engage in kriya yoga practices like kapalabhati.

49. SPEECH

Mauna

Speech is powerful.

In Hinduism, Sanskrit is understood to be a divine language. The words do not only represent objects; the sounds themselves are believed to contain the divine essence of the object they describe. Many traditions recognize speech as a creative power; the Old Testament begins, "In the beginning was the Word...and the Word was God."

Speech creates meaning. When we speak, we become creators with the capacity to both uplift as well as destroy. Consider the damaging power of gossip: once a rumor has been started, it's impossible to fully erase the story from our minds, even if it's untrue. In our modern world, our "speech" can include all the ways we may use words: emails, texts, and posts on social media.

We often forget about the power of our words and may use them carelessly.

Taking time to examine our relationship to speech can help us to become more mindful in our expression and be present in this moment. The practice of silence (*mauna*) can help us recognize the enormous amount of energy output that speaking requires. When we restrain our speech, we become aware of the impact our words can have. Practicing silence helps our minds to become calmer; we become more interested in taking in the world, rather than filling it.

PRACTICE

▶ Choose a time where you will be able to practice silence for at least a few hours, or even a day.

▶ Reflect on what practicing silence give you.

REFLECTION

▶ What is the quality of your speech?

▶ Why do you speak?

▶ Do you use speech to cover up discomfort (filling the silence, avoiding real communication or vulnerability)?

▶ Do you ever speak when you're not sure if someone else is interested?

▶ Practice being "impeccable with your word" (*The Four Agreements*, don Miguel Ruiz) and speaking only with integrity (*satya*) for one day. What is the result?

50. RITUALS

Vedas

Many cultures have used rituals to generate power, commune with natural and supernatural forces, and achieve transcendental states of insight. The rituals of Vedic culture (ancient Hinduism) included fire rituals, sacrificial rituals, and use of plant medicine.

A modern yoga practice has its own set of rituals: placing the mat to create a sacred space, becoming conscious of the breath and body, engaging in focus and discipline during the practice, death meditation *(savasana)*, and then the return to the world.

However, beyond our yoga practice, creating a personal ritual can support us in creating a framework of mindfulness for our day. We can use a ritual to set an intention, connect with our highest self, and steer our own course.

REFLECTION

Create a ritual that you can do each morning or each evening. Your ritual doesn't have to be long; even five minutes can help you create a mindful state.

Consider what you wish to create in your ritual. What activities or contemplations will help you reconnect to your self and your values?

Your ritual might include the following:

▶ Write or journal.

▶ List what you are grateful for.

▶ Do a brief asana practice to connect with your body.

▶ Consciously breathe or meditate.

▶ Set a written/spoken intention.

▶ Read an inspirational quote.

▶ Listen to inspirational or elevating music.

51. TAKING SPACE FROM THE WORLD

Pratyahara

Have you ever wished to just get away from it all?

The world is full of distractions, obligations, and stress. When we get pulled in every direction it's easy to lose our sense of groundedness, stability, and ease. Nourishing our introspective capacity is a vital act of self-care.

In *The Yoga Sutras*, Patanjali enumerates an eight-step process to yoga. Step five is *pratyahara*, or sense withdrawal. Part of the journey toward meditation and personal insight is to take a retreat from the distractions of the world.

In meditation, pranayama, or asana practice, this withdrawal effortlessly occurs as we become less interested in the outer world. You may have experienced this on your mat as your mind naturally becomes quieter and less restless during your practice.

Our senses—and our minds—are habituated to racing after what brings us pleasure, like coffee, chocolate, praise, or material acquisitions. When we become grounded in ourselves (sometimes just by taking 10 slow, conscious breaths), the clamoring of these compulsions begins to quiet. As the senses withdraw, we become less compulsive and attracted to objects in the outer world. As our inner sense of self begins to stabilize, we reconnect to our fundamental ground of being and presence.

REFLECTION

How can you support taking a personal retreat from the world?

Consider the following:

▶ Enjoy a daily meditation. Even two minutes can be nourishing.

▶ Withdraw from technology: turn off computers and phones for a designated length of time.

▶ Take time in nature.

▶ Take a weekend retreat.

▶ Embrace a daily "quiet time" practice.

▶ Give yourself permission to be unavailable to others.

▶ Create daily, uninterrupted, "self" time.

52. COMMUNITY

Kula

Your *kula* is your community, clan, or family. In yoga, a kula is your spiritual community, which comes together with a shared intention and purpose for growth and connection. Within our kula, we find a trustworthy support network to wrestle with spiritual questions and support one another through the challenges of daily life.

The yoga path can sometimes look solitary. After all, one chapter of *The Yoga Sutras* is entitled "Aloneness"! Kula reminds us that although our yoga path is often introspective and personal, we can choose to travel our path in very good company. When we connect to—or create—a community of like-minded souls, we have the opportunity to give and receive support for our highest intentions, and support one another in upholding our most precious values.

Seeking support on this path is a sign of wisdom.

REFLECTION

▶ Who do you consider part of your kula?

▶ Do you have new relationships you wish to nourish?

▶ What further communities/resources could support your path?

▶ How can you set time aside to nourish your heart connections?

*Yoga is about
doing funny shapes with
your body, simply for
the joy of being alive.*

We root to rise. What anchors you in your life? Today, nourish your roots to find your greatest expansion.

Open to grace.

Delight in discovering your edges.

Balance is
never fixed;
it is constant
recalibration.

Spanda: the divine vibration of the universe as it continually dances between expansion and contraction. Everything has a fundamental pulse: our heartbeat, the seasons, our feelings, even the planetary orbits.

Did you know…

The hatha yoga tradition is rooted in alchemy? Just as alchemists would try to transmute lead into gold, we are participating in a similar process of transmutation when we practice hatha yoga. While we may not literally become gold, we are metaphorically refining ourselves, becoming more lustrous, pure, and radiant from the inside out.

Dare to fall.

Self-discovery begins
at the edges of
your comfort zone.

Trees with the most magnificent branches also have the deepest roots.

Some of my best students
are inflexible.

I have often heard, "I can't practice
yoga, I'm not flexible enough."
However, flexible people often need more
strength building practices
to balance their natural mobility.
If you are stiff, a yoga class
is the perfect place to be.

POSES

90/90 POSE

▶ From a seated position on your mat, place your right leg directly in front of you with your knee flat on the ground. Be sure to keep your leg at a right angle. Repeat this motion with your left leg, moving it behind you.

▶ Slowly bring your chest down toward your knee, keeping your shoulders squared and remembering to breathe. Keep your elbows close to your body unless they can reach your mat evenly, then rest them on your mat. Hold for 20 to 60 seconds, or lean further forward to intensify the stretch, completing 6 to 10 repetitions of 3 seconds each.

ABDOMINAL TWIST
(Jathara Parivartanasana)

▶ Lie on your back and bring your knees up to your chest. Breathe for 3 rounds to help relax your lower back. Then, place your arms out to the side at shoulder height with your palms facing upward. Exhale, then bring your knees over to the right and up toward your right elbow.

▶ Stretch your left arm away from your legs to deepen the twist. Press your left shoulder blade into your mat to help anchor the stretch. Exhale, then twist your chest further to the left. Round your lower back slightly to pull the stretch through your spine. Hold for 30 seconds, then bring your knees back to center. Repeat on the opposite side.

Baby Cobra
(Ardha Bhujangasana)

▶ Lie prone on your stomach and bring your hands under your shoulders, keeping your elbows tucked close to your body. Press the tops of your feet firmly down and lengthen your tailbone toward your heels.

▶ As you inhale, straighten your arms to lift your chest off the floor slightly, keeping your pelvis and legs connected to the ground. Draw your upper arms back slightly and bring your chest forward into a small backbend. Take 3 to 5 deep breaths. Slowly lower your upper body to your mat, and then press back into **Child's Pose** (see page 17) for several breaths.

Bridge Pose
(Setu Bandha Sarvangasana)

▶ Lie on your back, bend your legs, and place your feet flat on the floor so that your ankles are just below your knees. Allow your arms to rest along your side, palms facing down, and tuck your elbows in by your ribs.

▶ On an inhale, lift your hips up, keeping your thighs parallel. Press your tailbone downward. Lift your chest upward. Press the back of your head lightly down to keep your gaze looking up. To deepen your backbend, interlace your hands beneath your hips and press your upper arms into your mat to lift your chest. Take 5 deep breaths. Release your hands and slowly roll down through your spine to lie flat, continuing to breathe. Repeat 2 more times.

Camel Pose
(Ustrasana)

▶ Kneel with your knees and feet hip distance apart. Tuck your toes. Press your tailbone back and downward with your hands on your lower back. Lift through your torso and draw your lower belly in and up and your shoulders back and down.

▶ Hinging from your hips, bend your upper body back to a comfortable degree. If you feel secure, lean back and grasp your heels. Keeping your chin tucked to your chest, lift your chest up and bend your upper back, keeping your thighs parallel. Press your pelvis forward and bring the curve through your spine. Honor the position that feels supported in your lower back and breathe. To come out, bring your hands to your lower back and bring your upper body back to upright.

Cat/Cow Pose

(Marjaryasana/Bitilasana)

▶ Begin on your hands and knees. Place your palms under your shoulders and set your knees under your hips. As you inhale, drop your belly toward the earth, reach your chest forward through your arms, and tip your lower back up to the sky.

▶ As you exhale, press through your hands, look toward your belly, and round your spine upward. Continue arching and rounding your spine to find length through the front and back of your body. Link your breathing with the movement, feeling your body open on the inhale, and contract on the exhale.

CHAIR POSE
(Utkatasana)

▶ Begin in **Mountain Pose** (see page 34). Bring your toes together and your heels slightly apart. Press your legs together.

▶ On an exhale, bend your knees, sink your hips back, and tuck your tailbone down, keeping your weight centered on your heels. Reach your arms forward and up and relax your shoulders down your back. Engage your core. Sit deeper into the pose to strengthen your legs, back, and core. Remain for 5 slow breaths, then stand and release your arms to your sides. Take a breath and enjoy the strength of your body.

CHILD'S POSE
(Balasana)

▶ Sit with your toes together and your knees a little wider than hip distance apart.

▶ Hinge forward from your hips to place your forehead on the earth or a block. Allow your arms to fall where feels comfortable. Check the position of your forehead against the floor and ensure that the skin of your forehead is wrinkling down toward the bridge of your nose rather than up. Let your face relax. Allow your head to get heavy and your belly to be soft and open. As you inhale, feel your breath move into your back ribs and lower back. As you exhale, allow any muscular tension to soften and let go. Remain in the pose for as long as feels nourishing. When you come out, take a few moments to stretch the backs of your knees by extending your legs back, or come into **Downward-Facing Dog** (see page 20).

Cobra Pose

(Bhujangasana)

▶ Lie prone on your stomach and bring your hands under your shoulders, keeping your elbows tucked close to your body. Press the tops of your feet firmly down and lengthen your tailbone toward your heels.

▶ As you inhale, straighten your arms to lift your chest off the floor, keeping your pelvis and legs connected to the ground. Draw your upper arms back and bring your chest forward. Walk your hands closer in under your shoulders, stretching through your legs. Take 3 to 5 deep breaths. Slowly lower your upper body to your mat, and then press back into **Child's Pose** (see page 17) for several breaths.

Corpse Pose

(Savasana)

▶ Lie prone on your back with legs extended. Turn your palms up and lay them a few inches from your sides or on your chest and stomach. Let your body fully relax. Close your eyes. Take several long, smooth breaths and release the tension from your body. Let your breathing slow down. Remain in this pose for a least 5 minutes.

▶ To come out, draw your knees into your chest and roll onto your right side. Cradle your head on your right arm and take a few breaths. When you're ready to sit, use your top hand to press yourself slowly to a comfortable seat. Take a few slow breaths.

Cow Face Pose

(Gomukhasana)

▶ Begin with your legs in front of you and your back straight, with your hands beside your hips. Bend your knees and bring your feet to rest on the floor. Bring your left foot under your right knee, then cross your right leg over your left, keeping your heels evenly apart from your hips. Rock slightly to balance your sitting position.

▶ Inhale and bring your right arm parallel to the floor. In one motion, rotate your arm so your palm faces the ceiling above your shoulder. Exhale and bring your right arm behind your torso, keeping your palm at the junction of your shoulder blades. Keep your right elbow parallel to your shoulder at all times. Repeat the circular stretching motion with your left arm, then bring your left arm behind your back and interlace your right and left hands. Lift your chest, hold for 1 minute, then reverse and repeat with your opposite leg on top.

You are not
a problem
to be solved.

You are
already whole.

Today, we are the driver who is irritated by the oblivious pedestrian. Tomorrow, we will be the pedestrian, irritated by the crazy driver! When we recognize that we almost always have been "the other guy" at one point or another, we can soften and remember that we're all on the same team.

Did you know…

"Hatha" actually means forceful? I like to remind my students of this fact when I hold them in plank pose for a long time.

It takes time to share love,
and we often rush
by our opportunities.
Pause for an extra
moment to share your
appreciation for someone.
Spread your love
outwards in little minutes.

Love is not only expressed in grandiose gestures.

Love is revealed
through our small,
daily acts of kindness.

Love is expressed
through the details.

Through relationships,
we discover ourselves.

Love is not to be
confused with surrender.
While love can be soft
and nurturing, love
can also blaze wildly
and fiercely.

Is it okay to fall asleep in Savasana?

Yoga confession: I have woken myself up out of Savasana with a ripe old snore. If you fall asleep in Savasana, do not fret. Your body simply needs the rest. Let go. Enjoy.

Love is our capacity
to expand, rather than
contract, when faced
with adversity.

Love means
softening rather
than hardening.

"May all beings everywhere be happy and free."

— MANGALA MANTRA

Downward-Facing Dog
(Adho Mukha Svanasana)

▶ Begin on hands and knees. Turn your hands so your index fingers point forward and spread your fingers wide. Press into your fingers to take weight off of your wrists. Curl your toes under and lift your knees slightly.

▶ Keeping your knees bent, send your hips toward the sky. Press your index knuckles down and your forearms toward each other, then press your upper arms upward to relax your neck. Keeping your spine long, straighten your legs. Stretch from your hands through to your heels. Take 5 to 10 deep breaths. On your last exhale, slowly lower your knees and sit your hips back on your heels to come into **Child's Pose** (see page 17).

Eagle Pose
(Garudasana)

▶ Stand in **Mountain Pose** (see page 34) with your hands on your hips. Bend your knees deeply to come into **Chair Pose** (see page 17). Press into your left foot and come onto the ball of your right foot. Turn your right knee inward about 45 degrees.

▶ From **Chair Pose**, lift your right leg as high as you can over your left thigh and squeeze the tops of your thighs together. Press your right shin into your left shin or wrap your right foot around your left calf. Lengthen your tailbone down, lifting your torso upward.

226

▶ Bring your arms wide, then wrap your arms. Hold on to your opposite shoulders or twine your forearms with palms together. Lift your elbows and press your forearms forward, opening your shoulder blades. Press into your standing foot, unwind your arms and legs, and release the pose. Repeat on the other side.

Easy Seat
(Sukhasana)

▶ Sit cross-legged, crossing at your shins. Switch legs so that your "non-traditional" shin is in front. Your shins should be placed far enough away that there is an open, triangular space between your hips and legs. Relax your legs fully. Rock slightly to find the center of your tailbone. Stretch your spine. Place your hands on your thighs and draw your arms back. Inhale and allow your ribs to expand. As you exhale, feel the subtle lifting of your pelvic floor. Soften your muscles, your face, and your eyes. Keeping the back of your neck long, tip your chin toward your chest until you feel a soft tension through the front of your throat, as if you were holding an orange beneath your chin. Your body is now ready to meditate.

Exalted Warrior Pose
(Viparita Virabhadrasana)

▶ Beginning in **Warrior 2** (see page 51), place your left palm on your left thigh. Turn your right palm upward and reach with your arm toward the ceiling. Deepen your backbend, being sure to support the stretch in your lower back. Tilt your chin upward to help relax your neck, being sure to push your shoulders back and down and keep your tailbone angled down.

▶ Maintaining your backbend, lean on your right knee, keeping your knee in line with your ankle. Hold for 5 to 10 breaths, then come out of the backbend and come up into **Mountain Pose** (see page 34).

Extended Cat Pose

(Utthita Marjaryasana)

▶ Starting in the center of your mat, come into **Tabletop Pose** (see page 47), keeping your hips aligned with your knees and your shoulders in line with your wrists. Keeping your neck relaxed downward, lean onto your left hand and extend your right arm forward, pointing your thumb toward the ceiling.

▶ Lift your stomach upward into a slight backbend and stretch your right leg behind you, with your toes resting on the ground. Once you feel comfortably balanced, lift your right toes off of the ground and stretch your leg out behind you. Be sure to keep your hips level and your shoulder blades stretched along your spine. Hold for 3 to 5 breaths, return to **Tabletop Pose**, and repeat on the opposite side.

EXTENDED CHILD'S POSE
(Utthita Balasana)

▶ Begin in **Child's Pose** (see page 17). Rest your weight on your heels and extend your arms up and over your shoulders, coming to rest with them in a triangle shape in front of you. Round your spine and slowly move downward until your forehead rests firmly on the ground and your fingers are either spread wide or on top of each other. Allow your body to fully relax into your mat, keeping your hips in contact with your heels. Hold for as long as feels nourishing. When you come out, take a few moments to stretch the backs of your knees by extending your legs back, or move into **Downward-Facing Dog** (see page 20).

EXTENDED HAND-TO-FOOT POSE
(Utthita Hasta Padangusthasana)

▶ Begin in **Mountain Pose** (see page 34). Then, bring your left knee up and toward your stomach. Move your left arm along the inside of your left thigh, then cross it over your left ankle and hold on to the outside of your foot. If this position is too tight on your hamstrings, you can use a strap around your foot.

▶ Press into your right leg and bring your left thigh inward. Inhale and extend your left leg outward. Straighten your knee as far as possible. You can stay here, or extend your leg out to the side if you feel balanced. Hold for 30 seconds, then bring your leg back to center on an inhale and to the floor on an exhale. Repeat on the opposite side, then return to **Mountain Pose**.

Eye of the Needle Pose

(Sucirandhrasana)

▶ Begin in **Hero's Pose** (see page 30), then recline onto your back. Cross your right ankle over your left knee and draw your left knee into your chest, keeping the back of your shin against your thigh. Breathe into the tightness of your outer hip and allow your right hip to settle toward your body. Close your eyes and let your head rest onto the floor. Take 10 deep breaths, then slowly change sides.

Finger Stand Cobra

(Bhujangasana, Variation)

▶ Begin on your stomach with your legs extended behind you and your feet flat on your mat, keeping your legs slightly apart and in line with your hips. Bring your hands out to either side of your chest, just past the edge of your mat. Bend your elbows so they point upward, then raise the palms of your hands until you are resting on the tips of your fingers in a claw-like position.

▶ Press your feet, legs, hips, and fingertips into your mat to support your body, then lift your head and chest upward. Pull your stomach inward and press your tailbone downward to support your body, arching your back as you do so. Lift your chest and head upward, dropping your shoulders back and outward as you do so to deepen your stretch. Straighten your arms almost all the way, keeping your elbows slightly bent. Hold for 3 to 6 breaths, then lower your torso back to the floor, focusing on your breathing.

Forearm Plank

(Phalakasana, Forearm Variation)

▶ Come to your hands and knees with your hands under your shoulders and your knees under your hips. Come down onto your forearms and step one foot back at a time. Lift your hips to the level of your shoulders, and then lengthen your tailbone back to your heels to engage your core and support your lower back.

▶ Lift your front ribs in as you draw your shoulder blades closer together and expand your chest. Press back through your heels as you reach your chest forward. After 30 seconds to 1 minute, lower your knees softly to your mat, press back into **Child's Pose** (see page 17), and take a few deep breaths.

Forward Fold

(Uttanasana)

▶ Stand with your feet hip distance apart and parallel. Inhale, roll your shoulders back, and lift your chest to lengthen your spine.

▶ As you exhale, bend your knees and hinge forward from your hips. If possible, bring your chest onto your thighs so that your upper body is supported by your legs. Fold forward as deeply as you can with a straight spine, allow your back to round, and release your head toward the earth. Take a few deep breaths, feeling the backs of your legs open and releasing any tension through your neck and jaw. Let your upper body hang heavy. To come out, relax your knees, bring your hands to your hips, and lift your shoulders. Press through your feet and slowly rise to stand.

Tapas: a Sanskrit word that describes the heat and friction necessary for change. Tapas is our willingness to endure intensity for the sake of transformation.

Clear your
space to clear
your mind.

❋ ❋ ❋

Showing up
is the most
important step.

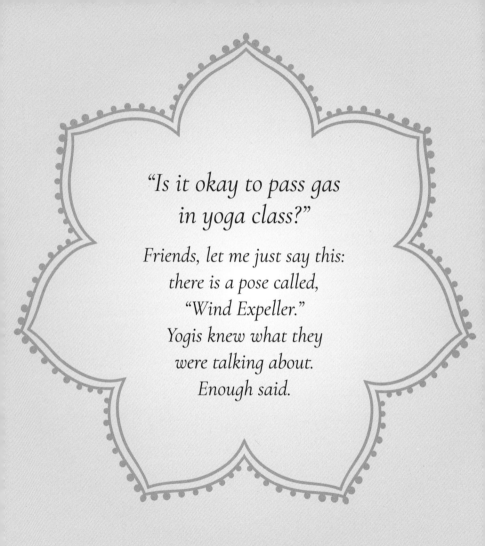

"Is it okay to pass gas
in yoga class?"

Friends, let me just say this:
there is a pose called,
"Wind Expeller."
Yogis knew what they
were talking about.
Enough said.

You are stronger
than you know.

Boundaries
create
freedom.

To many of us, boundaries seem harsh, as if they were an imposed separation or division. This is a confusion. Boundaries are loving and flexible membranes that are necessary for health and vitality. Think of our cells, discerning what will bring health and ease, and what will bring discord. In the same way, our capacity to hold mindful boundaries allows us to uphold a nourishing environment for both ourselves and for others.

"Do, or do not.
There is no try."

– YODA

Did you know…

Yoga is at least three thousand years old.

Let go of self-limiting beliefs.

Don't believe
everything
you think.

Lean into uncertainty.

Four-Limbed Staff Pose
(Chaturanga Dandasana)

▶ Begin in **Plank Pose** (see page 36). Push your shoulder blades back and down and angle your tailbone toward the front of your hips. Exhale, then lower yourself down until your body and legs are a few inches above the floor and parallel to your mat. Focus on keeping your tailbone level with the rest of your body, tensing your stomach to help lift your hips.

▶ Be sure to keep your shoulders stretched and your elbows close to your body. Pressing into your index fingers, lift the front of your chest upward and look forward. Hold for 10 to 30 seconds. Exhale, then either come to lay on your mat or shift back into **Downward-Facing Dog** (see page 20).

Frog Pose
(Mandukasana)

▶ Begin facing the long edge of your mat, then come into **Tabletop Pose** (see page 47). Walk your knees out to either side so they are wider than your hips. You should feel a deep stretch through the insides of your hips. If you feel any discomfort, bring your knees closer together.

▶ Turn your feet to either side, so they are perpendicular to the long edge of your mat. Move your heels directly behind your knees, and lean your arms and chest forward to come to rest on your forearms. If necessary, add a block under your forearms or hips to help support your body. Focus on stretching your head forward and angling your tailbone back. Your hips should stay above your knees to prevent undue strain. Lift your stomach in and back and hold this pose for up to 2 minutes. Move your knees back toward the center of your mat and come into **Child's Pose** (see page 17).

GODDESS POSE

(Utkata Konasana)

▶ Begin in **Mountain Pose** (see page 34). Then, turn toward the long side of your mat and bring your feet approximately 3 feet apart. Turn your heels in and your toes out, so your feet are at a 45-degree angle. Exhale, bend your knees, and bring your thighs parallel to your mat with your hips over your knees. Be sure your knees stay above your heels in order to feel the full effect of the stretch.

▶ Bring your arms out and to the side at shoulder height, then bend your elbows to right angles with your palms facing outward. Spread your fingers and bring your shoulder blades back and out. Tense your core and bring your lower ribs back and up. Center your tailbone over your hips, keeping your shoulders in line with your hips. Stretch through your heels and hold the pose for 5 breaths. To come out, stand upright, lower your arms, and return to **Mountain Pose**.

HALF SUN SALUTATION
(Ardha Surya Namaskar)

▶ Begin in **Mountain Pose** (see page 34). Make sure your back is fully stretched and relax your shoulders. Then, inhale and reach your arms outward and upward for **Upward Salute** (see page 49). Bring your palms together above your head or allow them to stay shoulder distance apart. Look upward to relax your neck.

▶ Exhale and bend your knees slightly into **Forward Fold** (see page 25). Allow your body to relax into the fold. Be sure to center on your feet, as leaning too far back can put undue strain on your hips.

▶ Inhale and come up into **Halfway Lift** (see facing page). Be sure to keep your spine flat by moving your hands to the most comfortable position on your legs.

▶ Exhale back into **Forward Fold**. If desired, rest here for 2 to 3 breaths to help fully release your spine.

▶ Inhale and rise up, reaching your arms back up for **Upward Salute** with your shoulders even and spread outward.

▶ Exhale and bring your hands to your sides to return to **Mountain Pose**. Repeat these poses 4 times, focusing on the connection of your movement with your breathing.

HALFWAY LIFT

(Ardha Uttanasana)

▶ Begin in **Forward Fold** (see page 25). Place your hands on either your shins or the floor in front of your feet. Inhale, straighten your arms, and unfold your torso outward as far as you can, creating a space between your pelvis and navel.

▶ Pushing down with your hands, lift your sternum up and forward. Bend your knees as you arch your back, allowing the stretch to move through your shoulders and over the curve of your back down to your waist. Keeping your eyes forward and your neck long, hold the position for a few breaths. Exhale and return to **Forward Fold**.

HAPPY BABY

(Ananda Balasana)

▶ Lying on your back, exhale and bend your knees to your stomach. Inhale, grabbing the outside of your feet and bringing them upward. If you have difficulty fully stretching your legs, you can use a strap to hold your feet. Open your knees slightly wider than your hips, keeping your shins perpendicular to the floor. Push your heels into your hands, pressing down with your hands to deepen the stretch. Hold for 5 breaths, then relax back to a lying position.

Hero's Pose
(Virasana)

▶ Stack one or two blocks on top of each other. Sit on the blocks so that your ankles hug the outside of the blocks and your thighs are close and parallel to each other. Adjust your sitting height as needed for comfort. Rock slightly to find the center of your tailbone. Place your hands on your upper thighs, with palms facing up or down. Draw your arms back to widen your collarbones. Inhale and feel your lungs and ribs expand. As you exhale, feel the subtle lifting of your pelvic floor. Soften your muscles, your face, and your eyes. Keeping the back of your neck long, tip your chin toward your chest until you feel a soft tension through the front of your throat, as if you were holding an orange beneath your chin.

High-Crescent Lunge

▶ Begin in **Downward-Facing Dog** (see page 20) and raise your right leg toward the sky.
▶ Step your right foot to your right thumb, keeping your feet hip distance apart. Place your hand on your front thigh and lift your torso up to come into a high lunge. Lengthen your tailbone downward and straighten your back leg, keeping your left heel lifted. Reach your arms up by your ears into a wide Y shape. Lift your chest forward and up for a gentle backbend. Hold for 5 deep breaths and feel your inner body expand and open. On your final exhale, slowly bring your hands to the floor, step into **Downward-Facing Dog**, and take a few breaths before repeating on the other side.

INTERRUPTED BREATHING EXERCISE
(Viloma Pranayama)

▶ Begin in **Easy Seat** (see page 21) or **Hero's Pose** (see page 30). Place one hand on your belly and one hand on your lower ribs. Take a full breath in and out to prepare. Take a modest inhale into your belly. Pause. Take a modest inhale into your lower ribs. Pause. Take a final inhale into your upper chest. Pause. Exhale all the way out. Repeat this for 6 rounds, then return to your natural breathing.

KNEES-TO-CHEST POSE
(Apanasana)

▶ Lying prone on your back, bend your right knee toward your chest, keeping your left leg straight. Place your hands under your knee, lacing your fingers. Flex your left foot toward you, stretching your hip. Hug your knee closer toward your armpit, relaxing your neck and shoulders. Pull your shoulder blades outward, stretching your upper back. Breathe deeply, lengthening your spine and drawing your tailbone downward. Release your hands, straighten your leg, and repeat on the other side.

Legs-Up-the-Wall Pose

(Viparita Karani)

▶ Sit about a foot away from the wall. Lie on your side and swing your legs up the wall. For tighter hamstrings, position your pelvis further from the wall. Take a position where your legs can comfortably relax. Keep your chin level with the floor, adding a book behind your head if needed. Allow your back to completely relax into the floor, and let your legs relax and settle into the wall. Remain for about 5 minutes. To come out, bend your knees first into your chest, then slowly roll to one side. Take your time to come up, and sit quietly for a few moments.

Locust Pose

(Salabhasana)

▶ Lie on your stomach with your arms at your sides, palms facing down. Press the tops of your feet firmly down, keeping your legs parallel. Lengthen your tailbone toward your heels. Roll your shoulders down your back and exhale.

▶ On an inhale, lift the whole length of your body, keeping your gaze down. Stretch your hands back toward your heels. Reach back through your toes, keeping your legs parallel. Focus on the length of the stretch instead of height. Stay for 3 breaths, breathing into your upper chest. On your last exhale, lower your body and release your hands. Turn your head to one side and completely let go. Repeat. After 3 rounds, take a few breaths and return to **Child's Pose** (see page 17).

Low Lunge
(Anjaneyasana)

▶ Begin on all fours with your hands just wider than your shoulders and your knees just behind your hips. Place your right foot by your right thumb. Bring your hands to your right thigh to lift your torso upward. Square your hips with your tailbone pointing down. Settle your hips forward and down to stretch the front of your left thigh. Be sure to keep your knee over your right heel.

▶ Draw your front ribs in and reach your arms forward and up in a wide V. Press your thighs together for stability. Draw your chest out into a mini backbend. Stretch through the length of your torso and out through your fingertips. Take 3 deep breaths. You can choose to keep your left knee down or lifted. As you exhale, bring your hands to your front thigh and then your mat. Step your right foot back, take a few breaths in **Child's Pose** (see page 17), and repeat on the other side.

Remember your own
magnificence.

Om.

When we chant Om, we are connecting to the source sound of the Universe.

Did you know…

For most of its long history,
yoga has been a practice
of meditation. Only in the past
hundred years has yoga become
so focused on postures.

Tat Tvam Asi:
You are That.

The yoga practice invites us to return again and again to the mat. Not for the sake of self-improvement, but to remove our confusion that we are not already whole.

"Our peak pose today,"
I said in one of my classes, "is
utthita hasta padangustasana."

I heard a student whisper:
"Is that a kind of pasta?"

Mountain Pose

(Tadasana)

▶ Stand with your feet either hip distance apart or together and parallel to each other. Lift your toes and stretch your inner and outer arches. Keeping your arches lightly stretched, relax your toes and press your feet downward. Engage the top of your thighs, with your tailbone pointing down and pelvis even. Draw your lower belly slightly in and up, then inhale and lengthen your waist. Roll your shoulders back and down and stretch your fingertips downward. Relax your front ribs in and down and draw your shoulder blades slightly together. Stretch your neck so your chin is level with the floor. Relax your eyes and take 5 to 10 deep breaths, becoming aware of the strength of your body.

Nesting Eagle Pose

(Garudasana, Variation)

▶ Begin in **Eagle Pose** (see page 20). Swing your left arm under your right and either hold on to opposite shoulders or twine your forearms and press your palms together. Take 2 deep breaths, then hinge from your hips to come forward with your elbows in front of your knees. Hold this pose for 5 to 10 breaths. To come out, lift your torso upward, untwine your arms, and untwist your legs, coming out into **Mountain Pose** (see above).

One-Legged Chair Pose

(Eka Pada Utkatasana)

▶ Begin in **Chair Pose** (see page 17). Hold for 4 breaths, making sure to keep your thighs down low and your body weight shifted to your heels. Bring your palms together in front of your chest. Keeping your weight on your left foot, bring your right foot up and cross your right ankle over your left knee. Your legs should form a triangle opening with your hips. Hold this pose for 3 to 5 breaths.

▶ To deepen the stretch, lean your chest forward until your hands rest on your right calf. Depending on your personal balance, you can continue to lean forward until your fingers touch the floor, or you can release your right leg to the floor to return to **Chair Pose** before coming out of the pose.

Pelvic Clock

▶ Begin by bringing your knees completely to one side. Roll over onto that side and come onto all fours with your knees under your hips. Place your elbows under your shoulders, interlace your hands, and move your hips in a big, lazy circle to open your lower back and your shoulders. Move in one direction for about 5 rounds, then change directions. To come out, move up onto all fours and either stand up or lean forward into **Downward-Facing Dog** (see page 20).

Pigeon Pose

(Eka Pada Kapotasana)

▶ Beginning on hands and knees, bring your right knee to rest on the floor behind your right hand. Angle your right foot toward the left side of your mat, stretching your hip and not your knee. Flex your foot to stabilize the pose.

▶ Slowly extend your left leg straight back until it rests on the floor. Lift your pelvis, squaring it to your mat. If your right hip raises, rest on a blanket or block. Exhale and slowly walk your hands forward. Bring your torso to rest on the floor, or rest on your elbows. Hold for 5 breaths. Walk your hands back to rest slightly wider than shoulder width. Lift your collarbones and inhale to return upright. Hold for 5 breaths, then move into **Child's Pose** (see page 17).

Plank Pose

(Kumbhakasana)

▶ Come onto your hands and knees with hands under your shoulders and knees under your hips. Press into your hands and step one foot back at a time. Lift your hips to the level of your shoulders, and then lengthen your tailbone back to your heels to engage your core and support your lower back.

▶ Lift your front ribs in as you draw your shoulder blades closer together and expand your chest. Press back through your heels as you reach your chest forward. After 30 seconds to 1 minute, lower your knees softly to your mat, press back into **Child's Pose** (see page 17), and take a few deep breaths.

Prone Corpse Pose

(Supta Savasana)

▶ Begin on your stomach with your hands at your sides and legs out behind you. Bend your right knee and bring it in line with your right hip. Move your arms above your head and turn your face to the right. Relax completely. Take at least 5 breaths, then change sides. If needed, you can add a blanket or block under your hips or head to make this pose more comfortable.

Pyramid Pose

(Parsvottanasana)

▶ Begin in **Mountain Pose** (see page 34) and breathe deeply. On an exhale, spread your feet about 4 feet apart. Raise your arms upward, pushing your shoulder blades back and down to extend the stretch. Position both feet to point forward. Exhale and turn your torso toward your front foot. Level your hips and arch your upper torso slightly to find your balance.

▶ On an exhale, hinge your torso toward the floor, bending at your hips. Bring your fingertips to the floor or on blocks. Stretch through your front thigh and relax your head toward the floor. Keeping your hips level, bring your torso closer to your thigh. Hold for 15 to 30 seconds, then rise on the inhale. Repeat on the other side.

Reclined Cow Face Pose
(Supta Gomukhasana)

▶ Lie on your back and cross your right knee over the left. Inhale and grasp your ankles. Exhale and draw your feet toward the floor on either side of your waist. If you cannot fully bring your ankles to the floor, you can rest them on blocks for added support. Hold for 10 to 15 breaths.

▶ Unwind, come back to a neutral pose on your back, then switch to the opposite side.

Reclined Hand-to-Foot Pose
(Supta Padangusthasana)

This pose works best with a strap or towel, and can be done with a folded blanket for support.

▶ Lie on your back with your legs extended. Rest your head on the floor or a folded blanket, keeping your spine even. Exhale, then bend your left knee and bring your left thigh to your chest. Hug your thigh to your stomach, pressing down through your right thigh and heel to deepen the stretch.

▶ Place the strap around the arch of your left foot, holding the ends of the strap in both hands. Inhale, straighten your knee, and press your left heel upward. Adjust your hands on the strap until your elbows are straight. Widen your shoulder blades outward, then press them into your mat, keeping your hands as high on the strap as you can. Be sure to keep your chest flattened toward your mat.

▶ To deepen your stretch, extend your leg from the heel upward until you feel a strong stretch through your body. If possible, bring your foot closer to your head to fully release your hamstrings. Hold this pose for 1 to 3 minutes, then repeat on the opposite side.

RECLINED MOUNTAIN POSE
(Supta Tadasana)

This pose requires blankets or blocks to support the body.

▶ Arrange 2 blocks or blankets with one at the top of your mat and one near the bottom with room for your feet. Sit in the center of your mat facing the short end. Be sure to give yourself enough support under your knees to take some of the stress of this pose off of your lower back.

▶ Recline back with your head on the top block or blanket and your knees bent over the lower prop. Bring your hands to rest on either side and allow a gentle backbend to come into your lower back. If desired, support your lower back with an additional blanket. Hold this pose for 5 to 10 minutes, then slowly come up to a sitting position or remove the props and come into **Corpse Pose** (see page 18).

Did you know…

Yoga is traditionally
taught one on one?
Group classes are
a modern phenomena.

The world provides us with
continual opportunities
for practice. When we find
ourselves in an emotional
reaction, the Universe is giving
us a wonderful opportunity
to simply pause and feel.
For a moment, practice letting
go of the story and become
aware of the sensations
of your body. Can you rest in
that space of just being?

There is only now.

The Bhagavad Gita is a treasured Indian epic about a hero, Arjuna, who finds himself on the field of battle, about to go to war with his kinsmen over the throne. Although Arjuna's claim to the throne is just, he collapses in despair because he does not want to fight his own family. His charioteer reveals himself to be a god, Krishna, who counsels Arjuna to do his duty and fight. Krishna calls this kind of mindful action karma yoga, or "skill in action."

Revolved Chair Pose
(Parivrtta Utkatasana)

- Begin in **Chair Pose** (see page 17). Balance back on your heels and bring your hands together in front of you with your palms facing each other. Inhale and stretch through your spine. Then, exhale and bend forward, twisting to the right side and looping your left elbow outside of your right thigh to provide additional balance.

- Press your palms firmly together to help stretch your shoulder blades. Keeping your knees closely together, lower your hips down slightly, being sure to maintain your balance throughout the pose. Hold for 3 to 5 breaths, then bend forward into **Forward Fold** (see page 25). Return to **Chair Pose** and repeat on the opposite side.

Revolved Lunge
(Parivrtta Anjaneyasana)

- Begin in **Low Lunge** (see page 33) with your right leg forward. Press your palms together at the center of your chest. Lift your left knee, bring your heel back, and press upward with your head, lengthening your spine.

- On an exhale, twist your torso toward your right leg. Keeping your palms together, rest your left triceps on your right thigh. Lengthen your spine as you inhale and twist deeper as you exhale. Hold this pose for 1 minute or reach one hand downward and the other toward the ceiling. To come out, unwind, place your palms on your mat, and step into **Downward-Facing Dog** (see page 20). Repeat on the opposite side.

Revolved Side Angle Pose

(Parivrtta Parsvakonasana)

▶ Begin in **Warrior I** (see page 50) with your left foot forward and your right foot back. Place your hands on your hips.

▶ Exhale, twist left, and bring your torso down. Place your right arm along the outside of your left knee with your hand on the floor or a block. Raise your left arm alongside your head and stretch, softening your stomach. Hold for 30 seconds to 1 minute, inhale, and return upright. Exhale to undo the twist. Repeat on the opposite side, then come into **Mountain Pose** (see page 34).

Saddle Pose

(Supta Virasana)

▶ Begin in **Hero Pose** (see page 30).

▶ With a back support prepared if needed, exhale and lower your lower back, leaning on your hands, then your forearms, and finally your elbows to support you. Then, place your hands behind your pelvis and release your lower back and upper thigh muscles. Allow yourself to fully recline onto the floor or the back support. If your ribs point upward, use your hands to press down on your ribs and lift your pelvis toward your navel, or adjust your support. If needed, you can add a blanket under your knees to lessen the strain on your hips. Keep your knees even with your hips to prevent strain as well. Hold for 30 seconds to 1 minute. To come out, press into your forearms and raise using the pressure on your hands, leading with your sternum until you return to **Hero's Pose**.

SIDE ANGLE POSE
(Parsvakonasana)

▶ Stand facing the long side of your mat. Lift your arms out to shoulder height and step so that your ankles are under your wrists. Turn your right leg so your right toes point to the short end of your mat. Align your right heel with the arch of your left foot and tilt in your left toes. Bend your right knee until it is over your ankle.

▶ Shift your hips back and place your right forearm on your right thigh. Press your knee toward your front foot and bring your tailbone down and back. Press your right forearm down and draw your right shoulder back. Sweep your left arm over your ear and turn your chest slightly upward. Stretch through the tips of your fingers. Hold for 5 breaths. To come out, press into your front heel and inhale to lift your torso up, straightening your legs. Repeat on the left side.

SKULL-SHINING BREATH
(Kapalabhati)

▶ To begin, sit either on the floor, on a block, or on the edge of a chair. Lift tall through your spine and reach your arms overhead in a wide V position. Take a deep inhale, then exhale fully. Inhale halfway, then begin a series of short, sharp exhales through your nose at a rate of about 1 to 2 per second. Allow your inhales to drop in naturally and keep your chest lifted and open. Exhale 25 times. Take a few natural breaths in and out to conclude the pose.

Sphinx Pose
(Salamba Bhujangasana)

▶ Begin lying prone. Press the tops of your feet firmly down and lengthen your tailbone toward your heels to engage your core.

▶ On an inhale, prop yourself up on your forearms with your elbows under your shoulders. If you feel any discomfort, walk your elbows further forward. Roll your shoulders back and down, pull your forearms toward you, and push your chest forward. Pull your bottom ribs in slightly to widen your back, and exhale. Take 3 to 5 deep breaths. Slowly lower your upper body to the earth, and then press back into **Child's Pose** (see page 17) for several breaths.

Standing Backbend
(Anuvittasana)

▶ Begin in **Mountain Pose** (see page 34) with feet hip distance apart. Pull up through your legs, stretching through them until your knees feel higher. Keep your tailbone angled downward while drawing your stomach up and back and your chest forward. Allow your shoulders to relax.

▶ Place your palms on the center of your lower back, with your fingers pointing downward. Draw your elbows back and toward each other. Inhale and focus in on your core. Exhale and bend your spine back, being sure not to exceed what feels comfortable. Adjust your neck so it is in line with your spine, or tilt backward and allow to relax. Hold for 3 to 5 breaths, focusing on relaxing your chest and deepening your backbend. To come out, inhale and return to **Mountain Pose** slowly, using your palms to help bring your spine to an upright position.

Standing Side Bend
(Parsva Urdhva Hastasana)

▶ Begin in **Mountain Pose** (see page 34). Inhale and sweep your arms upward, reaching to press your palms together. If your shoulders are too tight, stop when your arms are parallel to your shoulders. Stretch through your arms and neck, tilting your head upward. Bring your ribs down and in, reaching your tailbone downward. Lift your chest upward to stretch your belly and hold for 5 breaths.

▶ Tilt your pose, starting at your hips and curving your side. Reach your arms to the same side, curving your whole torso. Breathe for 5 breaths, then repeat on the other side.

▶ Come back to center, bring your arms out to the side, and tilt your torso down into **Forward Fold** (see page 25).

Standing Split
(Urdhva Prasarita Eka Padasana)

▶ Begin in **High-Crescent Lunge** (see page 30) with your right leg forward. Lean forward and bring your torso to rest on your right thigh. Place your hands on the floor on either side of your right foot or a block.

▶ Walk your hands ahead of your right foot, shifting your weight to your right foot. Inhale and straighten your right leg, lifting your left leg upward. To maintain your balance, keep your hips and knees squared toward the front of your mat. Focus on pulling the stretch evenly through your body and hold for 30 seconds to 1 minute. On the exhale, lower your leg and repeat on the other side.

Sun Salutation A

(Surya Namaskar A)

▶ Stand in **Mountain Pose** (see page 34) with your feet hip distance apart and parallel.

▶ As you inhale, reach your arms up to the sky into **Upward Salute** (see page 49).

▶ As you exhale, **Forward Fold** (see page 25) and bring your fingers to the earth.

▶ As you inhale, bring your fingertips to your shins, and lift halfway up into a mini backbend.

▶ As you exhale, place your palms to the earth shoulder distance apart and step back into **Plank Pose** (see page 36).

▶ As you continue to exhale, slowly lower halfway or fully down to the earth into **Four-Limbed Staff Pose** (see page 26).

▶ As you inhale, reach your chest forward and up into **Cobra Pose** (see page 18) or **Upward-Facing Dog** (see page 50).

▶ As you exhale, engage your core and reach your hips up and back to come into **Downward-Facing Dog** (see page 20). Take 5 deep breaths.

▶ After 5 exhales, step or walk your feet to the front of your mat. Inhale, bring your fingertips to your shins, and lift halfway up into a mini backbend.

▶ Exhale into a **Forward Fold** with your fingertips on the earth.

▶ Inhale, press through your feet, and reach your arms up into the sky for **Upward Salute**.

▶ Exhale and bring your hands to your sides to come back into **Mountain Pose**. Repeat up to 5 times, and feel your whole body expand in this moving meditation.

Sun Salutation B
(Surya Namaskar B)

▶ Begin in **Mountain Pose** (see page 34). Bend your knees, then inhale and reach your arms up to the sky for **Chair Pose** (see page 17).

▶ Exhale into **Forward Fold** (see page 25). On the inhale, come into **Halfway Lift** (see page 29).

▶ Exhale, step back into **Plank Pose** (see page 36), and lower down into **Four-Limbed Staff Pose** (see page 26).

▶ Inhale into a backbend, then exhale to **Downward-Facing Dog** (see page 20).

▶ Step your right foot to your right thumb, lower your back knee, if desired, and reach your arms up into **High-Crescent Lunge** (see page 30).

▶ As you exhale, lower your hands to the earth and step back into a vinyasa or into **Downward-Facing Dog** for 5 deep breaths.

▶ Step your left foot to your left thumb and inhale to rise up into **High-Crescent Lunge** on the other side, and repeat the sequence.

▶ At the end of your last exhale in **Downward-Facing Dog**, walk, step, or jump your feet forward.

▶ Inhale into **Halfway Lift**, then exhale into **Forward Fold**.

▶ Inhale and bend your knees into **Chair Pose**.

▶ Exhale into **Mountain Pose**. Repeat the sequence, including the side switch, two more times, focusing on linking your breathing with your movement.

SUPPORTED CHILD'S POSE WITH TWIST

(Parivrtta Balasana)

This pose requires blankets or other props.

▶ Begin in **Child's Pose** (see page 17) with your knees wider than your hips and two or more blankets stacked at the short end of your mat. Point your toes backward, then slide the blankets between your thighs to support your chest and hips.

▶ Lean back into your heels. Lift up partway, then thread your right arm underneath your left to wrap around the blanket. You can rest your head on a block or book, if desired. Take 5 breaths, then change sides.

TABLETOP POSE

(Bharmanasana)

▶ Begin on your hands and knees with your knees hip distance apart and your palms directly under your shoulders. Look down at your hands and flatten your back, stretching through your spine and focusing on keeping your body stable. Press into your palms to relax your shoulders down and back. Press your tailbone back to stretch your spine. Hold the pose for 1 to 3 breaths, then come down into **Child's Pose** (see page 17) or step back into **Downward-Facing Dog** (see page 20).

Dare to
increase your
capacity for
pleasure.

Did you know...

Some of the oldest yoga
texts are called Upanishads,
which means to "sit down near,"
reflecting the close relationship
of the teacher to the student.

Practicing self-care is like washing the steps of your own temple.

The mat is a space to nourish your unfiltered, authentic connection to yourself.

Come to
the mat. All of
you is welcome
here.

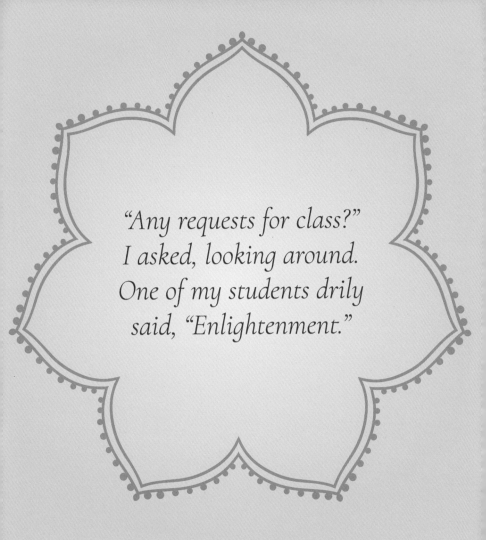

"Any requests for class?"
I asked, looking around.
One of my students drily
said, "Enlightenment."

Practice
radical
self-acceptance.

Be perfectly imperfect.

Take twenty minutes
just for you.

THREAD THE NEEDLE POSE
(Parsva Balasana)

▶ Begin in **Tabletop Pose** (see page 47), being sure your shoulders are above your wrists and your hips are above your knees. Inhale, then reach your right arm out and upward. Exhale and loop your right arm underneath your left arm. Lower your right shoulder and ear to your mat, stretching your right arm through the space created by your left arm to deepen the stretch.

▶ Be sure to balance your weight through your knees and feet, keeping your feet securely on your mat. Hold for 5 to 10 breaths, return to **Tabletop Pose**, and repeat on the opposite side.

THREE-LEGGED DOWNWARD-FACING DOG
(Eka Pada Adho Mukha Svanasana)

▶ Begin in **Downward-Facing Dog** (see page 20).

▶ Bring your left foot up and back, straightening your knee. Press back to feel the stretch, but do not over extend your hip. Keep your weight focused on your palms to help maintain your balance. Draw your tailbone back and your head forward toward the floor, bringing the stretch from your heel to your head. Hold for 5 to 10 breaths, then return to **Downward-Facing Dog** and repeat on the other side.

TREE POSE

(Vrksasana)

▶ Start near a wall or chair for added support. Stand in **Mountain Pose** (see page 34) and place your hands on your hips. Keeping your hands on your hips, press your left foot down and come onto the ball of your right foot. Turn your right knee out about 45 degrees. Place the sole of your right foot onto your left ankle, shin, or thigh above your knee.

▶ Press your foot into your standing leg. Lift from your torso to the crown of your head. Connect your palms together in front of your heart. If you feel steady, reach your arms overhead to enjoy a full stretch through the length of your body. To come out, bring your hands back together in front of your heart, turn your right knee forward, and then step your foot down. Repeat on the other side.

UPWARD SALUTE

(Urdhva Hastasana)

▶ Stand in **Mountain Pose** (see page 34) with your feet hip distance apart.

▶ Lift your arms up into a wide V above your head and stretch toward the sky through your fingertips, lengthening through the sides of your body. Relax the muscles at the base of your neck, draw your upper arms back by your ears, and open your chest. Breathe deeply. Stay in this pose for 2 minutes, continuing to stretch your whole body. After 2 minutes, relax your arms and take a few deep breaths.

UPWARD-FACING DOG

(Urdhva Mukha Svanasana)

▶ Lie prone on your stomach and bring your hands under your shoulders. Press the tops of your feet down to engage your legs. Lengthen your tailbone toward your heels, then lift your shoulders and roll them back.

▶ Press into your hands and lift your chest, then straighten your arms and lift your legs and pelvis off the floor. Press through the tops of your feet, relax your elbows, and press your chest forward, relaxing your upper arms. Lengthen the back of your neck. Take 3 breaths into your upper chest. To come up, draw your core in and up and lift your pelvis up and back to come into **Downward-Facing Dog** (see page 20). Lower your knees and come into **Child's Pose** (see page 17).

WARRIOR 1

(Virabhadrasana 1)

▶ Begin in **Mountain Pose** (see page 34) at the front of your mat.

▶ Step your left foot about 3 feet behind you. Position your left foot so it is at a 45-degree angle and your right foot points forward. Square your shoulders and hips toward the front of your mat. Bend your right leg until it reaches a right angle, aligning knee over ankle. Raise your arms upward and glide your shoulder blades down your back. Press your chest upward toward your raised arms. Arch your back slightly to find your balance. To come out, bring your arms to your sides as you step your left foot forward, breathing deeply into your opened chest. Repeat on the left side.

WARRIOR 2
(Virabhadrasana 2)

▶ Stand in the center of your mat and face the long side.

▶ Step your right foot forward and left foot back, about 4 feet apart. Keeping your hips and shoulders facing the long edge of your mat, bend your right knee so it is above your ankle. Align your right heel with the arch of your left foot, tilting your left toes inward so the outer edge of your left foot is parallel with the back of your mat. Lift from your pelvis and stretch through your torso. Ease your shoulders down and away from your ears, stretch your arms wide at shoulder height, and turn your head to look over your right fingertips. Take 5 slow breaths. Slowly straighten your right leg and turn your right thigh until parallel with your left. Lower your hands to your hips, inhale, and repeat on the left side.

WARRIOR 3
(Virabhadrasana 3)

▶ Stand facing the wall and place your fingertips on the wall at hip height. Make sure your hands are shoulder distance apart. Press your palms into the wall and step your feet back until your ankles are directly under your hips. Place your feet together and press your legs inward, bending your knees. Reach your hips back into the center of the room and stretch your spine fully, keeping your head directly between your arms.

▶ Keep your right leg straight and lift your left leg until level with your back, forming a T shape. Keep your hips square, stretching your inner left thigh upward and pushing your outer right hip back. Stretch fully through the length of your body and breathe. Slowly lower your left foot down to come back into an L shape. Repeat on the other side.

WIDE-LEGGED FORWARD FOLD

(Prasarita Padottanasana 1)

▶ Begin in **Mountain Pose** (see page 34). Exhale, place your hands on your hips, and spread your feet about 4 feet apart parallel to each other. With a straight torso, bend at the hips. Place your fingertips on the floor under your shoulders, keeping your torso parallel to the ground. Look toward the floor, keeping your neck straight.

▶ On an exhale, bend your elbows and torso to move into a full forward bend, walking your torso back and down using your hands. Rest your hands on the ground where comfortable. Let your head and neck relax down. Hold for 30 seconds to 1 minute. To come out, bring your hands under your shoulders, press your torso up, and, with hands on hips, step your feet back to return to **Mountain Pose**.

Take a deep breath.

At any given moment,
you're only one
slow breath away from
a new point of view.

Pause.

Close your eyes.
Connect to your breath.
When you open your eyes,
what can you see that you
have never seen before?
What is fresh to your
point of view?

Much of our suffering stems
from the simple confusion
that we are our thoughts.
We become identified
with our racing minds.

When we pause, we can
recognize that there
is a great space within us.
We are the Presence
watching our thoughts.

Did you know...

The irrigation of the nostrils with salt water—now prescribed by doctors for sinus issues— was described as a yogic cleansing technique over 500 years ago.

Take three
deep breaths.

Stretch like a cobra.

You are the
home you seek.

Slow
down
to feel.

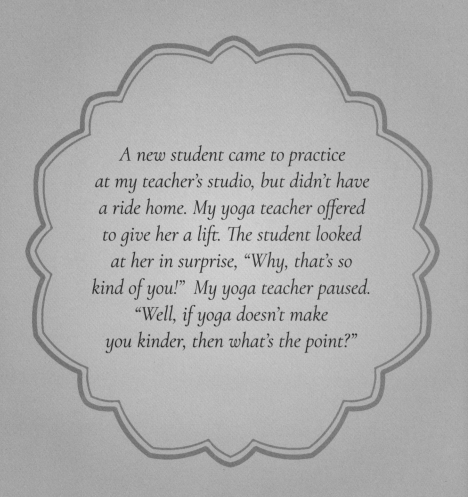

A new student came to practice
at my teacher's studio, but didn't have
a ride home. My yoga teacher offered
to give her a lift. The student looked
at her in surprise, "Why, that's so
kind of you!" My yoga teacher paused.
"Well, if yoga doesn't make
you kinder, then what's the point?"

Let go of the past,
let go of the future.
Now, allow your
body and your breath
to return you to this
present moment.

Shantih, shantih, shantih.
"Peace, peace, peace."

Sweet Morning Flow

▶ Come into **Extended Child's Pose** (see page 23) by bringing your hips back to your heels. Rest your forehead on your hands, a book, a block, or the floor. Gently roll your forehead side to side on the block to release any tension in your forehead.

▶ Keeping your left hip anchored back and down, walk your hands over to the right side of your mat for a side stretch. Take a few deep breaths to stretch your left ribs and the side of your body. Walk your hands back to center, then to the left and breathe into the right side of your ribcage.

▶ Come up onto all fours, placing your hands slightly wider than shoulder distance apart with your knees under your hips. Do 5 to 10 rounds of **Cat/Cow Pose** (see page 16). Move with the pose by shifting your hips side to side and continuing the spinal curve through your torso.

▶ Curl your toes underneath you and press up and back into **Downward-Facing Dog** (see page 20). Press into your hands as you bend your knees and stretch the tops of your thighs up and back. Take 5 deep breaths, and exhale through your mouth to release any tension in your throat and jaw.

▶ Walk your feet up to your hands, straighten your knees, and allow your upper body to release over your legs into **Forward Fold** (see page 25).

▶ After 3 breaths, bring your hands to your hips, lift your shoulders, and rise up into **Mountain Pose** (see page 34).

▶ Begin **Sun Salutation A** (see page 45). Stand in **Mountain Pose** with your feet hip distance apart and parallel. As you inhale, reach your arms up to the sky into **Upward Salute** (see page 49). As you exhale, **Forward Fold** and bring your fingers to the earth. As you inhale, bring your fingertips to your shins and move into **Halfway Lift** (see page 29).

▶ As you exhale, place your palms to the earth shoulder distance apart and step back into **Plank Pose** (see page 36). As you continue to exhale, slowly lower halfway or fully down to the earth into **Four-Limbed Staff Pose** (see page 26). As you inhale, reach your chest forward and up into **Cobra Pose** (see page 18) or **Upward-Facing Dog** (see page 50).

▶ As you exhale, engage your core and reach your hips up and back to come into **Downward-Facing Dog** (see page 20). Take 5 deep breaths. After 5 exhales, step or walk your feet to the front of your mat. Inhale, bring your fingertips to your shins, and lift halfway up into a mini backbend. Exhale into a **Forward Fold** with your fingertips on the earth. Inhale, press through your feet, and reach your arms up into the sky for **Upward Salute**. Exhale and bring your hands to your sides to come back into **Mountain Pose**. Repeat 3 to 5 times. Arrive back in **Mountain Pose** and bring your hands to your heart. Close your eyes and set an intention for your day.

Strong Start

▶ Beginning on all fours, place your forearms on the floor under your elbows, interlace your fingers, and step one foot back at a time to come into **Forearm Plank** (see page 25). Stay for 15 breaths. Lower your knees, place your hands slightly wider than shoulder distance apart, and lift your hips up and back into **Downward-Facing Dog** (see page 20). Stay for 5 breaths.

▶ Walk your hands to your feet, then rise up to stand in **Mountain Pose** (see page 34). Begin **Sun Salutation A** (see page 45). As you inhale, reach your arms up to the sky into **Upward Salute** (see page 49). As you exhale, **Forward Fold** (see page 25) and bring your fingers to the earth. As you inhale, bring your fingertips to your shins, and move into **Halfway Lift** (see page 29).

▶ As you exhale, place your palms to the earth shoulder distance apart and step back into **Plank Pose** (see page 36). As you continue to exhale, slowly lower halfway or fully down to the earth into **Four-Limbed Staff Pose** (see page 26). As you inhale, reach your chest forward and up into **Cobra Pose** (see page 18) or **Upward-Facing Dog** (see page 50). As you exhale, engage your core and reach your hips up and back to come into **Downward-Facing Dog**. Take 5 deep breaths.

▶ Reach your right leg up and back behind you. As you exhale, draw your right knee to your nose and into **Plank Pose** and pause. Inhale and reach your left leg back up into **Three-Legged Downward-Facing Dog** (see page 48), then draw your knee to your nose and stretch forward into **Plank Pose**. Reach your leg up and back into **Three-Legged Downward-Facing Dog**, then draw your knee to your nose and step your foot between your hands. Turn your back heel on its side and line up your front heel to your back arch.

▶ Windmill your arms up to **Warrior 2** (see page 51). Bend your right knee so that it is directly above your ankle and your front thigh is parallel to the floor. Press your left knee wide toward the right side of your mat so that you stretch your outer glute. Press into your back heel and straighten your left leg. Take 8 slow, deep breaths. Bring your hands to the floor and either step back into **Downward-Facing Dog** or take a vinyasa. Repeat this series, beginning with **Plank Pose**, on your left side.

▶ Inhale and reach your right leg up and back into **Three-Legged Downward-Facing Dog**. As you exhale, draw your right knee across your body to your left elbow. Repeat twice. On the third exhale, step your right foot to your right thumb. With your feet hip distance apart and parallel, inhale and reach your arms up to the sky for a **High-Crescent Lunge** (see page 30). Deeply bend your back knee and hover it off the floor as you stretch your arms up. Hold this pose for 10 breaths.

► As you exhale, take your hands to the floor, place your left hand under your left shoulder, and reach your right arm up to the sky to come into **Revolved Side Angle Pose** (see page 41). Stay for 5 breaths, lengthening on the inhale and twisting to your right as you exhale. Lower your hand and either step into **Downward-Facing Dog** or take a vinyasa. Repeat the lunge and twist on your other side. From **Downward-Facing Dog**, walk, step or jump your feet up to your hands. Inhale into **Halfway Lift**, and exhale into **Forward Fold**. Inhale and rise all the way up to stand, reaching your arms to the sky. Exhale and bring your hands to your heart for **Mountain Pose**. Close your eyes and take 5 slow, deep breaths, setting your intention for the day.

Satisfying Start

▶ Start on your back in **Reclined Mountain Pose** (see page 39) with your knees bent and your feet as wide as your mat. Drop your knees in toward each other and completely relax your hips. Take 10 deep breaths, feeling your body relax into the floor.

▶ Begin to move your knees from side to side slowly for a variation of an **Abdominal Twist** (see page 14) for about 5 rounds, relaxing your spine as you move.

▶ Begin **Pelvic Clock** (see page 35) by bringing your knees completely to one side. Roll over onto that side and come onto all fours with your knees under your hips. Place your elbows under your shoulders, interlace your hands, and take your hips in a big, lazy circle to open your lower back and your shoulders. Move in one direction for about 5 rounds, then change directions.

▶ Come onto your hands and begin **Cat/Cow Pose** (see page 16), arching and rounding your spine, for about 10 breaths.

▶ Curl your toes underneath yourself and press up and back into **Downward-Facing Dog** (see page 20). Inhale and come forward into **Plank Pose** (see page 36), then exhale back to **Downward-Facing Dog**. Repeat 5 times.

▶ Exhale and lower all the way to the floor. Place your fingers wider than your mat. Perch on your fingertips with your elbows straight above your wrists. As you inhale, draw your head forward and up for **Finger Stand Cobra** (see page 24). As your breathe, move freely, allowing one shoulder to drop forward and then the other, rolling your head and neck to help you fully relax your shoulder muscles. Stay for 5 breaths.

▶ Press up and back into **Downward-Facing Dog**. Walk your hands back to your feet, bend your knees, and bring your hands to your hips. Inhale and slowly lift up into **Mountain Pose** (see page 34). Bring your hands together in front of your heart and take 5 deep breaths to center yourself for the day.

QUICK START

▶ Bring your feet hip distance apart and parallel, bend your knees, and sit back into **Chair Pose** (see page 17). Bring your arms up at an angle, similar to a cactus. Tip your elbows forward slightly and your hands back. Then, claw the air with your fingers and pull down to feel your shoulder blades pull back and your chest lift forward and up. Take 10 breaths, widening your chest and pressing into your heels.

▶ Exhale and **Forward Fold** (see page 25), inhale into **Halfway Lift** (see page 29), then exhale and step back into **Plank Pose** (see page 36). Interlace your hands behind your back, then lift your chest forward and up for **Locust Pose** (see page 32). Tense your core to stabilize your lower back, then lift your legs if you are able. Stay for 5 breaths.

▶ Exhale and press up and back into **Downward-Facing Dog** (see page 20) for 5 breaths. Enhance your stretch by bending one knee and pressing into the opposite heel one side at a time.

▶ At the end of your exhale, walk, step, or jump your feet to your hands. Inhale into **Halfway Lift**. Exhale and **Forward Fold**, then inhale back to **Chair Pose** (see page 17).

▶ The next two steps are linked together for one side of the body. Sitting low, cross your left thigh over your right, squeezing your legs together for **Eagle Pose** (see page 20). Swing your left arm under your right and either hold onto opposite shoulders or twine your forearms and press your palms together. Take 2 deep breaths, then hinge from your hips to come forward into **Nesting Eagle Pose** (see page 34) with your elbows in front of your knees. Keeping your arms as they are, unwind your legs slowly and extend your left leg toward the back of your mat.

▶ Step into **High-Crescent Lunge** (see page 30). Ensure your feet are hip distance apart and parallel, then release your arms and stretch them upward. Lower into your legs, bring your front thigh to a 90° angle, then press up through the ball of your back foot. Press through your feet as your reach up through your arms for 5 breaths.

▶ As you exhale, bring your left hand to the floor under your left shoulder and reach your right arm up to the sky for **Revolved Side Angle Pose** (see page 41). Sweep your arm back by your hip and rotate your arm and shoulder in wide circles for 5 rounds. Place your hands on blocks directly under your shoulders. As you inhale, drop your hips forward for a lunge, then exhale and pull your hips back and bend your torso over your front leg. Move forward and back to stretch your hamstrings. Hold this pose for 5 rounds, gently moving your hips back and forth.

▶ Step forward to the front of your mat and inhale into **Halfway Lift**. Exhale and **Forward Fold**. Inhale to **Chair Pose**, and repeat this flow on the opposite side. Step forward to the front of your mat, bend your knees, and release the weight of your upper body down to the floor for **Forward Fold**. You can let your body sway or hold onto opposite elbows.

▶ Bring your hands to your hips, bend your knees, and slowly rise up into **Mountain Pose** (see page 34). Bring your hands together in front of your heart and set an intention for your day.

BREATH-INFUSED START

▶ Start in **Mountain Pose** (see page 34) with your feet hip distance apart and parallel. Bring your left hand over your heart and your right hand over your left and feel your heartbeat. Take 5 deep breaths into your chest. Lower your hands to your side and press down through your feet. As you inhale, reach your arms wide and up, press your palms together, and look up at your fingers. As you exhale, slowly drag your pressed palms down through the center of your body. At about your navel, interlace your hands and press your palms toward the floor. Follow your hands with your gaze. Repeat 5 to 10 times.

▶ Begin **Half Sun Salutation** (see page 28) by inhaling and reaching your arms up to the sky for **Upward Salute** (see page 49). Exhale and bend your knees slightly into **Forward Fold** (see page 25). Inhale into **Halfway Lift** (see page 29). Exhale back into **Forward Fold**. Inhale, rise up, and reach your arms up into **Upward Salute**. Exhale and bring your hands to your sides. Repeat 4 times, focusing on the connection of your movement with your breath.

▶ To begin **Sun Salutation B** (see page 46) with a high lunge, bend your knees, then inhale and reach your arms up to the sky for **Chair Pose** (see page 17). Exhale into **Forward Fold**. On the inhale, come into **Halfway Lift**.

▶ Exhale, step back into **Plank Pose** (see page 36) and lower down into **Four-Limbed Staff Pose** (see page 26). Inhale into a backbend, then exhale to **Downward-Facing Dog** (see page 20).

▶ Step your right foot to your right thumb, lower your back knee, if you desire, and reach your arms up into **High-Crescent Lunge** (see page 30). As you exhale, lower your hands to the earth and step back into a vinyasa or into **Downward-Facing Dog** for 5 deep breaths. Step your left foot to your left thumb and inhale to rise up into **High-Crescent Lunge** on the other side, and repeat the sequence.

▶ At the end of your last exhale in **Downward-Facing Dog**, walk, step, or jump your feet forward. Inhale into **Halfway Lift**, then exhale into **Forward Fold**. Inhale and bend your knees into **Chair Pose**. Exhale into **Mountain Pose**. Repeat the sequence, including the side switch, two more times, focusing on linking your breathing with your movement.

▶ Stand in **Mountain Pose** with your left hand on your heart and right hand over your left, feeling your heartbeat and your breathing. Take 3 deep breaths to set your intention for the day.

WARRIOR STRONG

▶ Stand in **Mountain Pose** (see page 34) in the middle of your mat, facing the long side. Bring your hands together in front of your heart, closing your eyes to bring your attention inward. Take 5 long, deep breaths. Bend your knees, sit your hips back, reach your arms forward and up, and come into **Chair Pose** (see page 17). Press your heels down and bring your inner thighs slightly back and down. Then, angle your tailbone down slightly to lift through your lower belly. As you send your hips back, stretch the sides of your waist. Then, stretch all the way through your fingertips. Stay for 10 breaths.

▶ Open your eyes and step your feet out wide. Rotate your right thigh, shin, and foot so that they they face the short side of your mat. Turn your back toes in slightly, then bend your right knee and move down into **Warrior 2** (see page 51). Lift your arms to shoulder height and stretch through your arms. Sit down onto your right thigh until it is parallel to the floor. Wrap your right glute underneath you as you bring your left thigh straight and press through your back heel. Stay here for 10 long, slow breaths, allowing the slow, strong burn of this pose to build your energy. Repeat on the other side.

▶ Turn both feet toward the long end of your mat and bring your hands onto your hips. Inhale to lift your chest, and as you exhale, hinge over your pelvis into **Wide Legged Forward Fold** (see page 52). You can either bring your hands to the floor (or blocks) for support, or interlace your hands behind your back and lift your arms to the sky to add a shoulder opening. Press into your feet as you work to straighten your legs and release your upper body. Stay for 5 breaths. Bring your hands to your hips, soften your knees, and inhale to rise up.

▶ Turn your right thigh and foot toward the short end of your mat again, and bring your left toes slightly in. Bend your right knee square (as in **Warrior 2**), then hinge from your pelvis to send your tailbone toward your back heel and bring your right forearm onto your right thigh for **Side Angle Pose** (see page 41). Keep your knee directly over the center of your foot by tensing your right glute, then, turn your pelvis and chest to the left and reach your left arm up to the sky. You can also keep your right elbow on your knee, bring your elbow to the inside of your knee, or hover your elbow above your thigh. Stay for 10 breaths. Repeat on your left side.

▶ Return to **Mountain Pose**, feeling the strength of your legs and your connection to the earth. Take 3 deep breaths to anchor yourself.

QUICK AND BREEZY FLOW

▶ Begin in **Mountain Pose** (see page 34). Bring your hands to your heart and take 3 deep, clearing breaths. Begin **Half Sun Salutation** (see page 28) by inhaling. Reach your arms up to the sky for **Upward Salute** (see page 49). Exhale into **Forward Fold** (see page 25). Inhale into **Halfway Lift** (see page 29). Exhale back into **Forward Fold**. Inhale, rise up, and reach your arms up for **Upward Salute**. Exhale and bring your hands back down to your sides. Repeat 4 more times.

▶ Move into **Sun Salutation A** (see page 45) with a flowing lunge and half split by inhaling and reaching your arms up to the sky. Exhale into a **Forward Fold**. Inhale and raise into **Halfway Lift**. Exhale and step your left foot back behind you and lower your back knee down. Keeping your hands on the floor (or on blocks) by your front foot, inhale and drop your hips forward. Lift your chest forward, exhale, and slide your hips back into a **Forward Fold** over your front thigh. Move between these two movements on your inhale, and exhale at least 5 times, enjoying the fluidity through your shoulders, spine, and hips.

▶ After 5 to 7 rounds, step back to the front of your mat, step your right foot back, and repeat through your opposite side. Exhale and step back into **Downward-Facing Dog** (see page 20).

▶ From **Downward-Facing Dog**, stretch your right leg back and up into **Three-Legged Downward-Facing Dog** (see page 48). Open your hips, bend your left knee, then draw your right knee into your belly and make five giant circles with your right knee to take your hip through its full range of motion.

▶ Stretch your right leg straight back and inhale. As you exhale, draw your knee into your nose and shift forward into **Plank Pose** (see page 36). Inhale and stretch your leg back into **Three-Legged Downward-Facing Dog**, then exhale and draw your knee to your nose. Inhale and stretch your leg back, exhale and draw your knee to your nose, and then place your right foot between your hands.

▶ Turn your back heel down parallel to the edge of your mat and rise up into **Warrior 2** (see page 51). Keeping your front knee over your front heel, inhale and reach your right arm up to side stretch into **Exalted Warrior Pose** (see page 22). As you exhale, shift your hips back, bring your right forearm onto your thigh, and sweep your top arm over your ear for **Side Angle Pose** (see page 42). Alternate between these two shapes for 5 to 7 rounds. On your final exhale, take your hands all the way to the floor, step back into **Downward-Facing Dog**, and repeat on your left side.

► Take your hands all the way to the floor. Inhale to step forward to the front of your mat and come into a **Halfway Lift**. Exhale into **Forward Fold**. Inhale to rise all the way up and stand with your arms overhead for **Upward Salute**, then exhale and bring your hands to your heart into **Mountain Pose**. Close your eyes and take 5 slow, deep breaths.

QUICK CORE CONNECTION

▶ Begin by lying on your back in **Reclined Mountain Pose** (see page 39) with your knees bent and your feet hip distance apart. Take a few deep breaths to clear your mind.

▶ Draw your knees into your chest for **Knees-to-Chest Pose** (see page 31) and slide your hands behind your head. Relax your shoulders, point your elbows up to the sky, and relax your head into your hands. Keeping your lower back pressed to your mat, bring your legs into **Tabletop Pose** (see page 47) with your knees above your pelvis and inhale. As you exhale, draw your left elbow toward your outer right knee. Inhale and come back to center with your head off the floor. As you exhale, twist your right elbow to your outer left knee. Repeat 10 times each side. Then, draw your knees into your chest and take a few deep belly breaths.

▶ Roll over onto one side and come onto your forearms and your knees to prepare for **Forearm Plank** (see page 25). Place your elbows under your knees with your hands interlaced, then step one foot back at a time to straighten your legs. Bring your lower ribs up into your body and press your shoulders away from your ears. Stay for 15 breaths.

▶ Come down onto your knees, place your hands under your shoulders, and press up and back into **Downward-Facing Dog** (see page 20) for 5 breaths.

▶ Inhale and lift your left leg high. As you exhale, draw your knee to your nose, shift forward, and round your spine. Inhale and stretch your leg back into **Three-Legged Downward-Facing Dog** (see page 48); as you exhale, shift forward and round your body. Repeat twice more, then step your right foot up to your right thumb and lower your back knee down.

▶ Bring your hands together at the center of your chest, inhale, then exhale and bring your left elbow to your outer right knee for **Revolved Side Angle Pose** (see page 41). If you want, you can lift your back knee up to deepen the pose. Inhale and lengthen, then exhale and twist for 5 rounds of breathing. As you inhale, untwist and bring your hands to the floor, then step back into **Downward-Facing Dog**. Repeat on your opposite side.

▶ Walk your feet to your hands. With your feet hip distance apart, hold your opposite elbows and **Forward Fold** (see page 25). Hold for 10 breaths. Then, release your arms and slowly roll up through your spine. Stand in **Mountain Pose** (see page 34) for 5 slow breaths.

WONDER WALL

For this practice, you will need a clear space at a wall. If you are using a mat, place the short end of your mat at the wall.

▶ Place your hands at hip height on the wall, and step back into an L-shaped variation of **Warrior 3** (see page 51). Ensure your hands are shoulder distance apart. Press into your hands, bend your knees slightly, and push your hips back into the center of the room to lengthen your spine. Keeping your spine straight, begin to straighten your legs and hold for 10 breaths. Then, walk your feet back toward the wall and stand up.

▶ Turn around with your back to the wall and place your feet about shin distance from the wall. Lean your hips back into the wall. Bend your knees and sit down into **Chair Pose** (see page 17). Press your heels straight down into your mat, being careful not to slide them forward. Reach your arms forward at shoulder height. Keeping your low ribs pressed back into the wall, press your shoulders back and reach your arms straight upward. Hold for 10 breaths, then lean forward to stand up.

▶ Turn to face the long side of your mat with your left foot at the wall. Place your feet wide apart for **Warrior 2** (see page 51). Turn your left toes forward slightly. From the top of your right thigh, rotate your front leg until your toes point toward the short end of your mat and your ankle, shin, and thigh are aligned. Keeping your back heel pressed against the wall, bend your right knee into a right angle. Press your feet apart as you reach your arms wide. Take 10 breaths, then switch sides.

▶ Place your hands at hip height at the wall again and return to the L-shaped pose variation of **Warrior 3**. Press your hands into the wall and keep your spine straight. Bring your legs together and reach your right foot back toward the center of the room. Keep your arms straight and your hips squared. Stay for 10 slow breaths on each side.

▶ Walk your feet slowly forward and rise up into **Mountain Pose** (see page 34). Take 5 breaths and feel how refreshed your hips and shoulders are.

REVITALIZE YOUR FEET

▶ Begin on all fours. Tuck your toes underneath you, then sit back on your heels for a toe stretch in **Hero's Pose** (see page 30). To decrease the intensity of the stretch, you can sit on a block or lift your pelvis up slightly. If possible, allow your body weight to sink down onto your heels, relaxing your front ribs in and your shoulders down. Bring your hands together in front of your heart and take 5 to 10 deep breaths.

▶ Exhale, come onto all fours, point your toes, and tap the tops of your feet to your mat. Begin 5 to 10 rounds of **Cat/Cow Pose** (see page 16) to open your shoulders and hips.

▶ Press up and back into **Downward-Facing Dog** (see page 20) for 5 to 10 breaths.

▶ Walk your feet to your hands and **Forward Fold** (see page 25). Hold for 5 breaths.

▶ Roll up into **Mountain Pose** (see page 34). Shift your weight side to side, then forward and backward to feel connected to the earth.

▶ Bring your feet together. Sit down deeply into **Chair Pose** (see page 17) with your weight in your heels, and bring your hands together in front of your heart. Squeeze your legs together. Keeping your knees and thighs pressed in, lift your left foot off the floor and balance on your right foot for 5 slow breaths. Repeat on the opposite side.

▶ Stand in **Mountain Pose** with your feet together and your hands on your hips. Use your hands to keep your pelvis squared forward, then turn your right thigh out and bring your foot to your shin or upper inner thigh for **Tree Pose** (see page 49). If you feel stable, reach your arms up overhead. Press down into your standing foot as you stretch up through the sides of your body. Take 5 breaths, then repeat on the opposite side.

▶ The next four poses are linked together in a flow. Bend you knees and sit back into a deep **Chair Pose**. Inhale to lengthen your spine. As you exhale, bring your left elbow to the outside of your right knee for **Revolved Chair Pose** (see page 40). Inhale to lengthen, exhale to twist. Maintaining your twist, keep your knees aligned. With your knees pressed together, lift your left foot off the floor. Press your chest forward as you slowly stretch your left leg back toward the back of your mat. Keep your upper body low.

▶ Step back into **Revolved Side Angle Pose** (see page 41). Pressing strongly into your feet, squeeze your legs together. Inhale and rise up into **High-Crescent Lunge** (see page 30). Hold for 5 breaths.

▶ Bring your hands to the floor, bend your front knee, and step forward into **Standing Split** (see page 44). Press into your right heel and begin to stretch your right leg straight. Stretch your left leg up and into the air, rolling your outer left hip down to keep your hips square. For an extra balance challenge, lift one or both hands off the floor and bring them to your right calf. Take 5 breaths.

▶ Press into your right foot, bend your right knee, and draw your left knee into your chest. Bring your hands together in front of your heart and begin to stand up. Cross your left ankle over your right knee and sit your hips back for **One-Legged Chair Pose** (see page 35). Press your hips back and your chest forward for 5 breaths. Stand up, release your foot to the floor, and come into **Mountain Pose**. Shake out your legs as needed. Then, repeat the series on your opposite side.

▶ Once finished, stand in **Mountain Pose** with your hands at your heart, feeling the connection of your feet into the floor. Take 5 deep breaths.

Open Your Hip Flexors

▶ Begin in **Mountain Pose** (see page 34). Bring your hands to your heart and take 5 to 10 deep breaths to transition your attention from thinking to feeling. Open your eyes. As you inhale, reach your arms up.

▶ As you exhale, come into **Forward Fold** (see page 25). Inhale to lift halfway up, then step your left foot back behind you so that your feet are hip distance apart. Place your hands on your front thigh and rise into **High-Crescent Lunge** (see page 30). Bend your back knee to lengthen your glutes and bring your stomach back. Keep your right hand on your front thigh and reach your left arm up and over your ear to come into a side stretch. Keeping your stomach stretched back and wide, straighten your back leg and reach through your arm. Stay for 5 to 10 breaths, stretching your left glute to open and relax the front of your hip. Bring your hands to the floor, step forward, then repeat on the opposite side.

► From the front of your mat, step your left foot back and lower your back knee down. Place your left hand wide and off your mat. Draw your left shoulder blade outward, up, and back turning your chest upward for **Low Lunge** (see page 33). Bring your right hand upward. Stretch the sides of your throat as you press your shoulder blades back and stretch your chest into a twist/backbend combination. Press your legs toward each other and allow your pelvis to relax forward. Bring your weight above your left knee, flex your foot, and bend your knee for a thigh stretch. If desired, reach back with your right hand to hold your foot. Hold for 5 to 10 breaths, then change sides and repeat. Step back and come into **Mountain Pose**.

▶ As you inhale, reach your arms up. As you exhale, come into **Forward Fold** (see page 25). Inhale to lift halfway up, then step your left foot back behind you so that your feet are hip distance apart. Again, come up into **High-Crescent Lunge**, but this time, bend your back knee and press your tailbone toward the floor. Keeping your right hand on your front thigh, draw your stomach back and relax your front ribs inward. Reach your left arm upward to add a side stretch up and over to the right side. Keeping your body pressed backward, stretch your back leg out straight. Take 5 to 10 breaths, using your exhale to draw your stomach in. Inhale and reach your arms up, exhale into **Forward Fold**, then step forward to the front of your mat and repeat on the opposite side.

▶ Sit on your shins with your toes together and knees wide to prepare for **Saddle Pose** (see page 41). If you have difficulty bending your knees, substitute a side-lying or standing quad stretch. Place your hands behind you and lift your tailbone up toward your shins. You can walk your hands back, bring your elbows onto a support behind you, or come down onto your forearms. Keep lengthening the front of your thighs toward your knees to stretch your quadriceps. Take 10 breaths.

▶ Lift your chest up and bring your hands in front of you. Place your hands slightly wider than shoulder distance apart and lift up and back into **Downward-Facing Dog** (see page 20) for 3 to 5 breaths to stretch the backs of your legs. Walk forward into **Forward Fold**, then slowly rise up into **Mountain Pose**. Place your hands together in front of your heart and take a moment to appreciate your legs and all the places they take you.

Open Your Hamstrings

This series requires a strap or a towel, some blocks, and a timer.

▶ Begin on your back in **Reclined Mountain Pose** (see page 39) with both knees bent. Take 5 long, slow breaths. Focus on the connection of your body to your mat. Draw your right knee into your chest and place a strap (or towel) around the ball of your right foot. Press your right hip into the floor and stretch your foot up to the sky for **Reclined Hand-to-Foot Pose** (see page 38). You can leave your left knee bent with your foot on the floor, or straighten your left leg and press your thigh and heel firmly down into the floor. Relax your shoulders down and allow your head to rest on the floor. Hold for two minutes, then switch sides.

▶ Roll over onto one side and rise up onto all fours. Press firmly down into your hands, then tuck your toes underneath yourself and lift your hips up and back for **Downward-Facing Dog** (see page 20). Bend your knees and press the tops of your thighs upward. Keeping your thighs pressing upward, stretch your heels down toward the floor, and slide the balls of your feet toward the back of your mat to come into **Plank Pose** (see page 36). Stay for 10 breaths.

▶ Step your right foot to the front of your mat between your hands. Walk your hands to the left side of your mat and turn both of your feet to the left for **Wide-Legged Forward Fold** (see page 52). Ensure that your feet are parallel to each other and bring your weight forward into the balls of your feet. Soften the backs of your knees as you lift through the backs of your legs. Release your upper body and head toward the floor. Stay for 10 breaths.

▶ Walk your feet toward each other until they are parallel and hip distance apart to come into **Forward Fold** (see page 25). Hold on to your opposite elbows and bend your knees so that your upper body can release toward the floor. Take 5 breaths, then switch the crossing of your arms. After 5 more breaths, release your arms to the floor and slowly roll up to stand. Stand in **Mountain Pose** (see page 34), bring your hands to your heart, and take 2 to 3 centering breaths through your whole body.

Open Your Shoulders

This series requires a strap or a towel at the front of your mat.

▶ Stand in **Mountain Pose** (see page 34) and take 3 to 5 deep, clearing breaths to make a transition from thinking to feeling. To begin **Sun Salutation A** (see page 45), inhale and reach your arms up into **Upward Salute** (see page 49). Exhale into **Forward Fold** (see page 25), then inhale into **Halfway Lift** (see page 29). As you exhale, step back into **Plank Pose** (see page 36) and lower all the way to the earth. You can keep your knees straight if you wish. Inhale into a backbend like **Baby Cobra** (see page 15) or **Upward-Facing Dog** (see page 50), then exhale into **Downward-Facing Dog** (see page 20). Take 5 breaths.

▶ Inhale, step to the front of your mat, and come into **Halfway Lift**. Exhale into **Forward Fold**. Inhale, stand up, and reach your arms up into **Upward Salute**. Exhale and bring your hands to your sides. Repeat 2 to 4 times, focusing on the movement of your arms and breath. On your last round, stay in **Downward-Facing Dog**.

▶ From **Downward-Facing Dog**, step your right foot to your right hand so that your feet are hip distance apart and parallel. Using the strap, rise up into **High-Crescent Lunge** (see page 30). Bend your back knee slightly so that you can bring your tailbone downward. Hold the strap behind your back with your palms facing forward and your hands about shoulder distance apart. Relax your front ribs in slightly and draw your shoulders back. Keeping your core tensed, press your shoulders outward and stretch your arms back behind you. Continue to pull the strap apart as you reach your chest forward and up. Take 5 to 10 deep breaths into your upper chest to stretch your shoulders. Release the strap, bring your hands to the floor, and step forward. Then, step your right foot back and repeat on the second side. When finished, step back into **Downward-Facing Dog**.

► From **Downward-Facing Dog**, step your right foot to your right hand so that your feet are hip distance apart and parallel. Using the strap, rise up into **High-Crescent Lunge**. Bend your back knee slightly to stretch your tailbone downward. Reach your left arm up to the sky. Use your right hand to pull your left arm forward, then bend your left elbow and bring your hands to the middle of your back for a triceps stretch. If you are more flexible in your shoulders, you can bring your hand to your left shoulder blade. Use your right hand to bring your left arm in. Press your left shoulder back and out as you stretch through your left elbow. Take 5 breaths. Release your hands to the floor, step back into **Downward-Facing Dog**, then repeat on the opposite side.

▶ Step to the front of your mat into a **Forward Fold** and interlace your hands behind your back. If you need more space for your shoulders in the stretch, hold the strap between your hands. Bend your elbows, lift your shoulders up, and stretch your hands upward. Focus on keeping your shoulders lifted. Your elbows can remain bent with your palms apart. If you have more shoulder flexibility, you may eventually straighten your elbows and press your palms together. Take 5 deep breaths. Roll up slowly into a standing position.

▶ Inhale and reach your arms out wide. As you exhale, cross your arms in front of you with your right arm under your left and hold onto your opposite shoulders. Stay here, press the backs of your forearms into each other, or wrap your forearms and press your palms together like in **Eagle Pose** (see page 20). You can also bend your knees, rotate your right thigh inward, and lift and cross your right thigh over your left, pressing your shins together. Lift your forearms up and press them slightly forward to stretch your shoulders. Stay for 5 breaths, then unwind your arms and legs and switch sides.

▶ Stand in **Mountain Pose** with your feet hip distance apart. Hold the strap slightly wider than shoulder width apart. For this exercise, you can allow your hands to slide apart as far as you need on the strap, but keep your arms straight. As you inhale, lift your arms overhead. As you exhale, make a giant circle through your shoulders to bring your arms back behind you. Then, inhale and pull the strap apart as you lift your arms back upward. Exhale and bring your hands to your sides. Repeat 4 times. Stand in **Mountain Pose** and take 3 to 5 breaths, appreciating the openness in your chest, ribs, and shoulders.

Open Your Outer Hips

▶ Begin in **Easy Seat** (see page 21) with your shins crossed and your feet under your knees. You may wish to sit on a block, book, or pillow to lift your hips. Use your hands to press your glutes wide and slightly back in order to sit upright on your tailbone. Bring your hands to your heart and take a few centering breaths.

▶ Bring your fingertips behind you. Inhale and lift your chest. As you exhale, come into a **Forward Fold** (see page 25) over your cross-legged seat. If you can easily lengthen your chest forward, bring your hands in front of you and allow your spine to relax forward and down. Let your head relax and feel the stretch through your outer hips. Take 10 deep breaths. On your next inhale, rise up, change which shin is in front, and repeat on the opposite side.

▶ Begin on all fours for 5 rounds of **Cat/Cow Pose** (see page 16). Curl your toes underneath yourself and press backward into **Downward-Facing Dog** (see page 20). Hold for 3 to 5 breaths.

▶ Step your right foot between your hands, turn your left heel down parallel to the back of your mat, and rotate your arms upward into **Warrior 2** (see page 51). As you press your left thigh straight, press your right hip down toward the floor and press your right knee outward to stretch your right glute. Hold for 10 breaths. Rotate your hands down to the floor and step back into **Downward-Facing Dog**. Repeat on the opposite side.

▶ Sit on the floor and bring your right shin parallel to the front edge of your mat. Bring your back shin parallel to the left long edge of your mat, keeping each leg at a right angle and inhale. As you exhale, fold forward over your front leg for a variation of **Pigeon Pose** (see page 36). Keep your right hip pressed on the floor. You can adjust the angle of your front shin by moving your knee wider to the right or left, as well as adjust the angle of your body. If you can keep your right hip down, you may also slide your left foot back toward the back of your mat to increase the stretch on the front outer hip. If you feel any knee pain or pressure, discontinue this pose and opt for **Eye of the Needle Pose** (see page 24) instead. Hold for 20 breaths, then change sides.

▶ As you come out, sit on your left hip. Move your left knee slightly toward the center of your mat so that your knee is now in line with your pubic bone rather than your outer hip. Swing your right leg forward and bring it up and over your left leg, stacking your knees for **Cow Face Pose** (see page 19). Your hips should remain grounded and your ankles should be near your hips. It is okay if your knees are not completely crossed, so long as your knees feel comfortable. If you are having trouble, sit on a block or attempt the pose in a reclined position. Inhale to stretch upward. Exhale and fold forward and hold for 20 breaths. Straighten your legs, then repeat on the opposite side.

Mobilize Your Spine

▶ Begin in **Extended Child's Pose** (see page 23) with your knees wide, your hips on your heels, and your upper body relaxed toward the earth. Take 5 deep breaths to center yourself. Keeping your hips on your heels, walk your hands toward the right side of your mat for a lateral spinal stretch. Take 5 deep breaths, then move to the opposite side.

▶ Inhale, rise up onto all fours, and come into **Cat/Cow Pose** (see page 16), feeling the stretch through your whole body After a few rounds, explore different movements in the pose, such as rolling through your shoulders and shifting your hips from side to side.

▶ Curl your toes underneath yourself and lift your hips up and back into **Downward-Facing Dog** (see page 20). Press firmly into your hands, bend your knees, and stretch your hips upward. Push your thighs up and back, simultaneously reaching your chest outward toward your thumbs to lengthen your stomach. Hold for 10 breaths.

▶ Inhale and come into **Plank Pose** (see page 36). As you exhale, lower down into **Locust Pose** (see page 32). Stretch both your legs back hip distance apart and press the tops of your feet down. Roll your inner thighs upward and stretch your tailbone back to your heels. Reach your arms behind you and interlace your hands. Feel free to keep your hands free if interlacing them causes strain on your shoulders. Lift your shoulders upward, pressing them outward as you lift. As you inhale, lift up through your chest and legs, draw your hands toward your heels, and relax your chest forward. Take 3 breaths, focusing on stretching your back with every inhale. Lower down, then repeat 2 times.

▶ Prop yourself up on your forearms so that your elbows are under your shoulders for **Sphinx Pose** (see page 43). If you have any lower back discomfort, move your elbows further forward so that your lower ribs can stay on your mat. Stretch your tailbone back. Press your forearms down and pull your palms back to open your chest and widen your collarbones. For a deeper backbend, lift your elbows and continue to move your chest forward and up. Stay for 5 breaths, drawing your upper back forward and opening your chest as you inhale. Lower your body to the earth and look to one side.

▶ When you are ready, press up and back into **Downward-Facing Dog**. Then, step your right foot between your hands. Lower your back knee down. Place your hands at the center of your chest. Inhale to lengthen your chest, and as you exhale, twist to the right to place your left elbow outside your knee for **Revolved Lunge** (see page 40). You may leave your back knee down, or lift it for stability. Remain for 5 breaths, focusing on your spinal stretch. Then, lower your hands, move back into **Downward-Facing Dog**, and change sides.

▶ Step forward to the front of your mat. Bend your knees and hinge forward into **Forward Fold** (see page 25), allowing your upper body to relax fully. Remain for 5 breaths, then take 3 slow breaths to roll up through your spine to a standing position. Stand in **Mountain Pose** (see page 34), bring your hands to your heart, and take 5 slow, deep breaths.

Quick Wake Up

▶ To begin **Skull-Shining Breath** (see page 42), sit either on the floor, on a block, or on the edge of a chair. Lift tall through your spine and reach your arms overhead in a wide V position. Take a deep inhale, then exhale out fully. Inhale halfway, then begin a series of short, sharp exhales through your nose at a rate of about 1 to 2 per second. Allow your inhales to drop in naturally and keep your chest lifted and open. Exhale 25 times. Take a few natural breaths in and out.

▶ The next two poses are linked. To begin **Half Sun Salutation** (see page 28), inhale to lift your arms up into **Upward Salute** (see page 49), then exhale into **Forward Fold** (see page 25). Inhale into **Halfway Lift** (see page 29), then exhale and step your left foot back for a long lunge with your feet hip distance apart and parallel. If desired, lower your back knee. Bring your hands together in front of your heart. Inhale, lengthen your upper body, and exhale and twist to the right for **Revolved Side Angle Pose** (see page 41), bringing your left elbow outside your right knee. Take 3 breaths.

▶ Inhale to untwist and place your hands on either side of your front foot. If desired, lower your back knee. Pull your hips back, straighten your front leg, and fold forward into a variation of **Pyramid Pose** (see page 37). Take 3 breaths. If desired, flex your front foot and pull your toes upward. Bend your front knee and step forward, then repeat on your opposite side.

▶ Stand in **Mountain Pose** (see page 34) and take 3 deep breaths.

Quick Spinal Decompression

▶ Begin on all fours, then curl your toes underneath yourself and lift your hips up and back into **Downward-Facing Dog** (see page 20). Bend your knees and draw the tops of your thighs up and back. Keeping your hips lifted, press strongly into your inner hands and reach your chest toward your thumbs to lengthen both sides of your waist. If desired, bend a knee or press back into your heel to stretch your calves. You can also shift both heels from right to left and back again to stretch your waist.

▶ Walk your hands back to your feet, bend your knees, and allow your upper body to hang over your lower body into **Forward Fold** (see page 25). Turn your head side to side to release your neck. Sway side to side to release tension in your spine, if desired, bending your knees several time to help relax your whole body.

▶ Keeping your head and arms completely relaxed, slowly roll up through your spine over the course of 4 to 5 breaths, shifting your weight to your feet. If you become lightheaded, **Forward Fold** once more and move slower until your body can equalize. Once you come into **Mountain Pose** (see page 34), roll your shoulders up, back, and down several times to relax your neck.

▶ Place your hands on a wall shoulder distance apart with your hands at at hip height and step back into an L-shaped pose to come into a variation of **Warrior 3** (see page 51). Press into your hands, bend your knees slightly, and pull your hips back toward the center of the room to lengthen your spine. Keeping your spine straight, hug your feet and legs together, and begin to straighten your legs. Keeping your arms straight and your pelvis square to the floor, reach your right leg back toward the center of the room for 5 breaths. Lower your right leg, then lift your left leg for 5 breaths. Keep your arms and legs straight. Lower your leg, stand up, take a few deep breaths, and appreciate your newly relaxed body.

INSTANT DE-STRESS

▶ To begin **Half Sun Salutation** (see page 28), inhale and reach your arms upward for **Upward Salute** (see page 49). Exhale, bend your knees slightly, and **Forward Fold** (see page 25). Inhale and come into **Halfway Lift** (see page 29). Exhale back into **Forward Fold**. Inhale and reach your arms upward. Exhale and move your hands to your sides. Repeat 3 times, focusing on connecting your movement to your breathing.

▶ Come up into **Mountain Pose** (see page 34) with your hands over your heart. Feel your heartbeat. Inhale for a count of 4, then exhale for a count of 6. Pause between each breath. Repeat 5 times.

One Minute Unwind

▶ To begin **Legs-Up-the-Wall Pose** (see page 32), lay on your back with your legs against the wall. If you have tight hamstrings, position your pelvis 1 to 2 feet from the wall. You can also use a strap or tie a scarf around your thighs so that your legs can completely relax.

▶ Place one hand on your belly and one hand on your lower ribs. Take a full, complete breath in and out to prepare for a breathing exercise. To begin, take a modest inhale into your belly. Pause. Take a modest inhale into your lower ribs. Pause. Take a final inhale into your upper chest. Pause. Exhale all the way out. Repeat this for 6 rounds, then return to your natural breathing. When you're ready, slowly roll over onto one side and sit up.

HAPPY HEART OPENER

▶ Start in **Mountain Pose** (see page 34) and take 3 deep breaths. Reach your arms up overhead, turn your right palm upward, and hold onto your right wrist with your left hand. Relax your shoulders and press your tailbone downward. Lean into your right foot and curve your left side up and over to the left into an arch, bending at the waist. To deepen this side stretch, lift your left foot. Hold for 3 breaths, then change sides.

▶ Inhale and reach your arms up, then exhale into **Forward Fold** (see page 25). Inhale to come into **Halfway Lift** (see page 29), then exhale and step your left foot back. Rise up into **High-Crescent Lunge** (see page 30). Interlace your hands behind your head and point your elbows forward to relax your shoulders outward.

▶ Balance back onto your legs, keeping your weight centered over them. Press your chest back, tense your left glute, and straighten your back leg. Press your head into your hands and reach your chest forward and up. Take a deep breath. Lean into the ball of your back foot and push your front heel down to lift your stomach up. Tense your core as you exhale, then inhale to reach your arms straight upward. On your next exhale, press into your feet and bring your hands to the floor. Step forward, come into **Forward Fold**, and take 3 breaths. Step your right foot back and repeat **High-Crescent Lunge** on the opposite side.

As you step to the front of your mat, inhale and come into **Halfway Lift**. Bring your hands to your hips, then inhale and stand up. Place your hands on your heart in **Mountain Pose** and hold as long as feels nourishing.

CONCLUSION

"The nature of practice
is continual, devoted,
and for a long time."

—Sutra 1.14

Now that you have begun to use some of these concepts and tools, continue to explore how they can guide and support your work, play, and relationships. And be patient: yoga is a practice for a lifetime (or, according to the yogis, several lifetimes!) and we will often need to learn its lessons again and again.

Living our yoga is an invitation to stay awake, aware, and curious. When our minds create stories or we feel reactive, yoga asks us to perk up and lean in. Rather than live on autopilot, we can do our best to stay open to the freshness of this moment. Through this practice, we can start to experience the world as it is, rather than living through the lens of our assumptions and expectations.

INDEX

ABOUT THE AUTHOR

A yoga teacher, mentor, and educator, Rachel Scott helps teachers and studios around the world to create teacher trainings and continuing education programs. Her extensive knowledge and experience include earning two masters degrees, authoring three books, and leading over 4,000 hours of teacher training. As a writer and speaker, she continually wrestles with the juicy bits of life: relationships, authenticity, and discovering meaning in this crazy, wonderful world. She holds an E-RYT 500, YACEP, BA, MFA, and MSci and is a wicked coffee drinker. Learn more at rachelyoga.com.

About Cider Mill Press
Book Publishers

Good ideas ripen with time. From seed to harvest, Cider Mill Press brings fine reading, information, and entertainment together between the covers of its creatively crafted books. Our Cider Mill bears fruit twice a year, publishing a new crop of titles each spring and fall.

"Where Good Books Are Ready for Press"

Visit us on the web at
www.cidermillpress.com
or write to us at
PO Box 454
12 Spring St.
Kennebunkport, Maine 04046